Overview Map Key

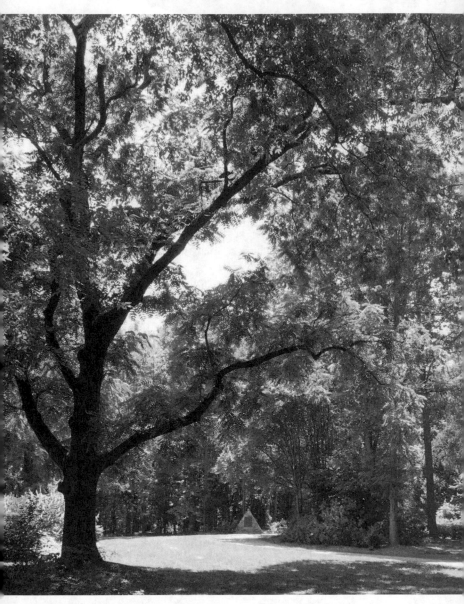

NEARLY 4 MILES OF TRAILS WIND ALONG THE LAKESHORE AND THROUGH THE FORMAL GARDENS OF BEAUTIFUL JETTON PARK.

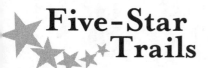

Five-Star Trails

Charlotte

Your Guide to the Area's Most Beautiful Hikes

Joshua Kinser

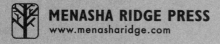

MENASHA RIDGE PRESS
www.menasharidge.com

Five-Star Trails Charlotte
Your Guide to the Area's Most Beautiful Hikes

Edited by Amber Kaye Henderson
Cover design by Scott McGrew
Text design by Annie Long
All photographs by Joshua Kinser unless otherwise noted
Cartography and elevation profiles by Joshua Kinser and Scott McGrew
Indexing by Rich Carlson

Library of Congress Cataloging-in-Publication Data

Kinser, Joshua.
  Five-star trails : Charlotte : your guide to the area's most beautiful hikes /
Joshua Kinser.
     p. cm.
  Includes index.
  ISBN-13: 978-0-89732-888-3
  ISBN-10: 0-89732-888-4
  1. Hiking—North Carolina—Charlotte—Guidebooks. 2. Trails—North
Carolina—Charlotte—Guidebooks. 3. Charlotte (N.C.)—Guidebooks. I. Title.
  GV199.42.N662C55 2012
  796.5109756—dc23
                                        2012030982

Menasha Ridge Press
P.O. Box 43673
Birmingham, AL 35243
menasharidge.com

Disclaimer
This book is meant only as a guide to select trails in and near Charlotte, North Carolina, and the greater metropolitan area. This book does not guarantee hiker safety in any way—you hike at your own risk. Neither Menasha Ridge Press nor Joshua Kinser is liable for property loss or damage, personal injury, or death that result in any way from accessing or hiking the trails described in the following pages. Please be especially cautious when walking in potentially hazardous terrains with, for example, steep inclines or drop-offs. Do not attempt to explore terrain that may be beyond your abilities. Please read carefully the introduction to this book, as well as further safety information from other sources. Familiarize yourself with current weather reports and maps of the area you plan to visit (in addition to the maps provided in this guidebook). Know park regulations, and always follow them. Do not take chances.

Contents

South of Charlotte   129

West of Charlotte   163

Appendixes & Index   205

Dedication

This book is dedicated to Jessica Nile. Thanks for being there with me every step of the way.

Acknowledgments

Thanks to all the trail crews and workers who have spent countless days in the dirt of the forest chipping rock, cutting trees, cleaning trails and rivers, and constructing bridges so that those of us who enjoy nature so much may have a path in which to explore it. Thanks also to those who have advocated for the trails and greenways around Charlotte. The trails are some of the best in the country, and creating them is no easy task. Your work does not go unnoticed or unappreciated. Finally, thanks to Susan Haynes and Scott McGrew for making the book possible, and to my friends and family for being so supportive of this project.

—*Joshua Kinser*

Preface

When I first started working on this project, I always got the same response when I told people who didn't live in Charlotte that I was writing a hiking guidebook to the city: *"Charlotte?* I didn't think there was much hiking in Charlotte." This couldn't be further from the truth, and those of us who live in and around this great city know how much hiking Charlotte has to offer. Truly amazing and diverse hiking experiences are here for the seeking.

True enough, most hikers and outdoor enthusiasts consider the Smoky Mountains region of the Appalachians to be the real jewel of Western North Carolina. But driving from Charlotte to Asheville and the national park isn't something you're going to do when you want to take a walk after work or spend a weekend afternoon hiking a leafy path alongside a rolling creek. And you don't need to, either. The mountains are a lot closer than you think: within an hour's drive from downtown. And so much hiking is available around Charlotte that you just can't experience anywhere else, so there's really no need to *go* anywhere else.

One interesting aspect about Charlotte is that no particular area around the city stands out as the epicenter of hiking. The best trails lie in every direction and they are spread out, so no matter where you live in Charlotte, or no matter where you're staying while you're visiting, you're likely to find a great trail nearby if you know where to look. This book makes it easy. It's divided into regions that include downtown Charlotte and the regions east, west, south, and north of town. Simply flip to the table of contents and check out the trails in the region closest to you.

If you're unsure where to start in your hiking explorations, then look no further than page xii of this book for a list of recommended hikes grouped in nine categories. The trails in this book have been selected to not only provide a selection of the best hikes in the city but also to provide a reflection of the different types of trails, routes, terrain, and environments you can experience around Charlotte. All of the trails in the book are day hikes and are offered in a variety of multiple lengths and varying difficulty, from a short and flat walk through a forest and around a pond on one of Charlotte's many great greenway trails to an arduous 7-mile foray into a mountainous wilderness.

In putting this book together, I made sure that it offered more than rugged trails through long trudges of mountains and gaps. I wanted this book to offer routes through every aspect of Charlotte. That's why it includes walks through downtown that let you explore key attractions, parks, and dining districts; a route through

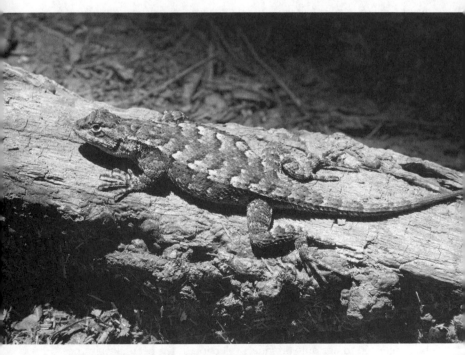

AN EASTERN FENCE LIZARD SUNBATHES BESIDE THE TRAIL AT LATTA PLANTATION.

the amazingly restored Historic Fourth Ward neighborhood, where you can take in the city's finest 19th-century homes; and detailed routes through two of the country's best botanical gardens: the University of North Carolina at Charlotte Botanical Gardens and the Daniel Stowe Botanical Garden. While the above are not challenging walks in the woods, they are just as memorable and really give you the opportunity to experience Charlotte as a whole and not just its parks and forests.

Die-hard hikers have no need to worry, though: I've included plenty of day-long ambles over rocky-topped mountains that get the heart racing and the calves pounding and take you to awesome vistas with views for miles. For these types of readers, the challenging hike to Shoal Falls, an 80-foot waterfall in South Mountains State Park, would be a great place to start (see page 66).

It is my hope that the book offers the right types of trails for many different types of people, and that it reaches an audience that is interested in exploring all of the hiking and walking experiences that Charlotte has to offer. In a time when so many folks seem to be increasingly disconnected from the outdoors, I'm proud to share these amazing trails. I hope this book will get people outdoors hiking or walking, and in the process contribute to their overall mental and physical well-being.

Whether you're a local or a visitor, I hope you'll use this guidebook to make some discoveries as well as visit some old favorites. Also, most of these trails are surrounded by other trails and outdoor destinations that are definitely worth exploring. So don't just stick to the routes I've written about here. Get out on your own and explore Charlotte's trails, greenways, parks, and walking routes, and find your own favorite five-star trail.

Recommended Hikes

Best for Wildlife

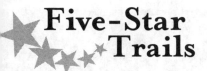

Five-Star Trails

Charlotte

Your Guide to the Area's Most Beautiful Hikes

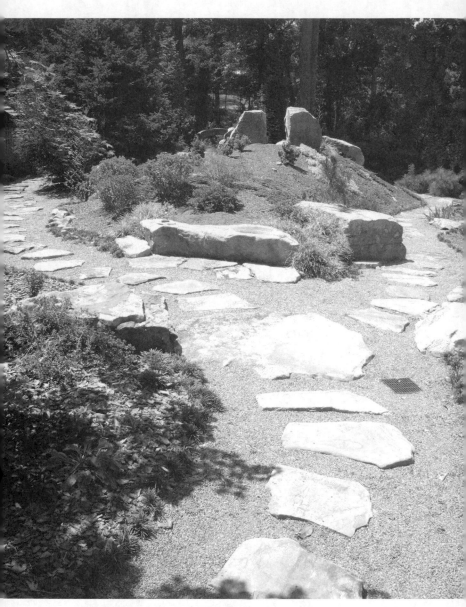

AN ARTFULLY CONSTRUCTED TRAIL WINDS THROUGH THE ROCK GARDEN AT
UNC CHARLOTTE'S BOTANICAL GARDENS.

Introduction

About This Book

Five-Star Trails: Charlotte provides route details, maps, elevation profiles, and photographs for 32 of the best hikes in this city and the surrounding region. Charlotte offers urban hikes in the heart of downtown as well as a variety of paved and unpaved greenways that spread out around the greater metro area. Those routes connect neighborhoods, parks, business districts, and green spaces for residents and visitors alike. Surrounding Charlotte is a variety of terrain ranging from mountains and Piedmont foothills to flatlands and small natural prairies.

While none of the hikes in this book get five stars in every ratings category, each will have one, two, three, or four stars in one or more of them. A hike might merit inclusion in this book because its scenery is spectacular, while another hike with two-star scenery is selected because it's considered five-star when it comes to taking children along. The star-rating system offers a simple and quick way to find the type of trail that's right for you.

Greater Charlotte's Geographic Divisions

The hikes in this book encompass five geographic regions. Each region has its own particular attraction, and they include star destinations such as urban greenways, South Mountains State Park, Crowders Mountain State Park, Uwharrie National Forest, McDowell Nature Preserve, the Latta Plantation, and much more.

Center City covers the urban core. Most of the hikes here utilize Charlotte's greenway system—one of the longest and most developed in the United States. Downtown and much of the metro area offer level topography, compared with the land around it, offering easy strolls through the city, parks, and leafy neighborhoods. These routes are best for short strolls and for nature trails through urban areas and small parks.

1

North encompasses the most diverse landscapes in the book. Many of the trails in this region are centered near or on Lake Norman. Or take an easy day hike on a mostly level greenway through University Research Park. An hour to the northwest, as you get closer to the Great Smoky Mountains National Park, you find dramatic mountain terrain, rocky creeks, and waterfalls in South Mountains State Park.

East includes the University of North Carolina at Charlotte area, where you'll find an easy stroll through the university's botanical gardens. Within the Charlotte Beltway, Reedy Creek Nature Preserve is just far enough north of the city to have hilly terrain. As you head farther west in this eastern section, the terrain becomes more mountainous, and you will find great hiking in Morrow Mountain State Park and in the 50,640-acre Uwharrie National Forest.

South stretches down to Waxhaw, North Carolina, and includes trails around the towns of Fort Mill, North Carolina, and Lake Wylie, South Carolina, in the entries for Cane Creek Park, McAlpine Creek Park, and McDowell Nature Preserve. The terrain is less challenging in this region than in many others. But these trails are especially good for light hiking, running, and after-work or short day excursions.

West covers the area from Mount Holly, North Carolina, just beyond the Charlotte Beltway, to Blacksburg, South Carolina. Similar to the North region covered in this book, the West region becomes increasingly more mountainous as you get closer to the main ridge of the Appalachian Mountains. Here more than any region herein, you can experience a variety of trails, including the historic and fascinating monuments and farms in Kings Mountain National Military Park and State Park and the outdoor-adventure complex of the U.S. Whitewater Center, where you can not only hike and bike the hilly trails but also raft down rapids on a man-made river and fly down high-elevation zip lines through a beautiful forest. All the way to the west, Crowders Mountain State Park has mountain terrain and challenging trails in a park bordering the Yadkin River.

How to Use This Guidebook

The following information walks you through this guidebook's organization to make it easy and convenient for planning great hikes.

Overview Map, Map Key, & Map Legend

The overview map on the inside front cover shows the primary trailheads for all 32 hikes described in this book. The numbers shown on the overview map pair with the map key on page i. Each hike's number remains with that hike throughout the book. Thus, if you spot an appealing hiking area on the overview map, you can flip through the book and find that area's hikes easily by their sequential numbers on the first page of each hike profile.

Trail Maps

In addition to the overview map on the inside cover, a detailed map of each hike's route appears with its profile. On each of these maps, symbols indicate the trailhead, the complete route, significant features, facilities, and topographic landmarks such as creeks, overlooks, and peaks. A legend identifying the map symbols used throughout the book appears on the inside back cover.

To produce the highly accurate maps in this book, I used a handheld GPS unit to gather data while hiking each route and then sent that data to the expert cartographers at Menasha Ridge. Of course, your GPS is really no substitute for sound, sensible navigation that takes into account the conditions that you observe while hiking.

Further, despite the high quality of the maps in this guidebook, the publisher and myself strongly recommend that you always carry an additional map, such as the ones noted in each profile opener's "Maps" listing.

Elevation Profile (Diagram)

For trails with significant elevation changes, the hike description will include this graphical element. Entries for fairly flat routes, such as a lake loop, will *not* display an elevation profile. Also, each hike description's opener lists the elevation range from the start of that specific route to the hike's highest point.

For hike descriptions that include an elevation profile, this diagram represents the rises and falls of the trail as viewed from the side, over the complete distance (in miles) of that trail. On the diagram's vertical axis, or height scale, the number of feet indicated between each tick mark lets you visualize the climb. To avoid making flat hikes look steep and steep hikes appear flat, varying height scales provide an accurate image of each hike's climbing challenge. For example, one hike's scale might rise 800 feet from the trail's start, while another might rise 160 feet from that start.

The Hike Profile

Each profile opens with the hike's star ratings, GPS trailhead coordinates, and other key at-a-glance information—from distance and configuration to contacts for local information. Each profile also includes a map (see "Trail Maps" on previous page). The main text for each profile includes the Overview, Route Details, Nearby Attractions, and Directions (for driving to the trailhead area). Explanations of each of these elements follow.

STAR RATINGS

Five-Star Trails is the title of a Menasha Ridge Press guidebook series geared to specific cities across the United States, such as this one for Charlotte. Following is the explanation for the rating system of one to five stars in each of the five categories for each hike.

FOR SCENERY:

★ ★ ★ ★ ★   Unique, picturesque panoramas

★ ★ ★ ★   Diverse vistas

★ ★ ★   Pleasant views

★ ★   Unchanging landscape

★   Not selected for scenery

FOR TRAIL CONDITION:

★★★★★ Consistently well maintained

★★★★ Stable, with no surprises

★★★ Average terrain to negotiate

★★ Inconsistent, with good and poor areas

★ Rocky, overgrown, or often muddy

FOR CHILDREN:

★★★★★ Babes in strollers are welcome

★★★★ Fun for any little one past the toddler stage

★★★ Good for young hikers with proven stamina

★★ Not enjoyable for children

★ Not advisable for children

FOR DIFFICULTY:

★★★★★ Grueling

★★★★ Strenuous

★★★ Moderate—won't exhaust you, but you'll know you've been hiking

★★ Easy, with patches of moderation

★ Good for a relaxing stroll

FOR SOLITUDE:

★★★★★ Positively tranquil

★★★★ Spurts of isolation

★★★ Moderately secluded

★★ Crowded on weekends and holidays

★ Steady stream of individuals and/or groups

GPS TRAILHEAD COORDINATES

As noted in "Trail Maps" (see page 3), I used a handheld GPS unit to obtain geographic data and sent the information to the cartographers at Menasha Ridge. In the opener for each hike profile, the coordinates—that is, the intersection of latitude (north) and longitude (west)—will orient you from the trailhead. In some cases, you can drive within viewing distance of a trailhead. Other hiking routes require a short walk to the trailhead from a parking area.

You will also note that this guidebook uses the degree–decimal minute format for expressing GPS coordinates. The latitude–longitude grid system is likely already quite familiar to you, but here's a refresher, pertinent to visualizing the coordinates:

Imaginary lines of latitude—called *parallels* and spaced approximately 69 miles apart from each other—run horizontally around the globe. The equator is established to be 0°, and each parallel is indicated by degrees from the equator: up to 90°N at the North Pole, and down to 90°S at the South Pole.

Imaginary lines of longitude—called *meridians*—run perpendicular to lines of latitude. Longitude lines are likewise indicated by degrees. Starting from 0° at the Prime Meridian in Greenwich, England, they continue to the east and west until they meet 180° later at the International Date Line in the Pacific Ocean. At the equator, longitude lines also are approximately 69 miles apart, but that distance narrows as the meridians converge toward the North and South poles.

To convert GPS coordinates given in degrees, minutes, and seconds to the degree–decimal minute format, the seconds are divided by 60. For more on GPS technology, visit **usgs.gov.**

DISTANCE & CONFIGURATION

Distance notes the length of the hike round-trip, from start to finish. If the hike description includes options to shorten or extend the hike, those round-trip distances will also be factored here. Configuration defines the trail as a loop, an out-and-back (taking you in and out via the same route), a figure-eight, or a balloon.

HIKING TIME

A general rule of thumb for the hiking times noted in this guidebook is 1.5 miles per hour. That pace typically allows you plenty of time for taking photos, for dawdling and admiring views, and for alternating stretches of hills and descents. When you're deciding whether or not to follow a particular trail in this guidebook, consider your own pace, the weather, your general physical condition, and your energy level on a particular day.

HIGHLIGHTS

Waterfalls, historic sites, or other features that draw hikers to this trail are emphasized here.

ELEVATION

In each trail's opener, you will see the elevation at the trailhead or other starting location and another figure for the peak height you will reach on that route. For routes that entail significant inclines and declines, the full hike profile also includes a complete elevation diagram (see page 3).

ACCESS

Fees or permits required to hike the trail are detailed here—and noted if there are none. Trail-access hours are also shown here.

MAPS

Resources for maps, in addition to those in this guidebook, are listed here. (As previously noted, the publisher and myself recommend that you carry more than one map—and that you consult those maps before heading out on the trail to resolve any confusion or discrepancy.)

FACILITIES

Alerts you to restrooms, water, picnic tables, and other basics at or near the trailhead.

WHEELCHAIR ACCESS

Tells you whether paved sections or other areas exist where persons with disabilities can safely using a wheelchair.

COMMENTS

Here you will find assorted nuggets of information, such as whether or not dogs are allowed on the trails.

CONTACTS

Listed here are phone numbers and website addresses for checking trail conditions and gleaning other day-to-day information.

Overview, Route Details, Nearby Attractions, & Directions

These four elements make up the heart of the hike. "Overview" gives you a quick summary of what to expect on that trail; "Route Details" guide you on the hike, start to finish; "Nearby Attractions" suggests appealing adjacent sites, such as restaurants, museums, and other trails. "Directions" will get you to the trailhead from a well-known road or highway.

Weather

In Charlotte, you can experience all four seasons. Enjoy these variations, but always give careful consideration to weather and prepare accordingly—especially when heading into mountainous areas to the north, west, and east of the city.

As a Southern city, Charlotte can get brutally hot in the summer—just the right time to head for higher, cooler ground in the surrounding mountainous areas. Summer also can bring afternoon thunderstorms, so it's often best to hike in the morning or evening, not only to beat the heat but also to avoid exposure to seriously dangerous lightning.

Spring and fall are long and mild and are the best times for hiking anywhere in and around the city. Spring weather can be volatile, however: a warm, beautiful, sunny day can turn into a cold and rainy one in a matter of hours. Visitors flock to the most popular trails in the fall, as the leaves begin to turn and display their colors. During these peak seasons, you should consider hiking early in the morning or during weekdays to avoid crowds.

Winter brings the city comparatively mild temperatures that only occasionally drop below freezing. The same can't be said for the higher elevations surrounding Charlotte, though—there you'll encounter frigid, below-freezing temperatures and occasionally snow, sleet, and hail. So plan accordingly in terms of attire and, very importantly, in terms of time: winter daylight hours are short, especially if you are hiking in forested areas.

The following chart lists average temperatures and precipitation by month for the Charlotte region. For each month, "Hi Temp" lists the average daytime high, "Lo Temp" lists the average nighttime low, and "Rain or Snow" lists the average precipitation. Expect cooler temperatures in the higher elevations, especially those in South Mountains and Morrow Mountain state parks.

MONTHLY WEATHER AVERAGES FOR CHARLOTTE, NORTH CAROLINA			
MONTH	HI TEMP	LO TEMP	RAIN OR SNOW
January	51°F	30°F	3.41"
February	55°F	33°F	3.45"
March	63°F	39°F	4.01"
April	72°F	47°F	3.04"
May	79°F	56°F	3.18"
June	86°F	65°F	3.74"
July	89°F	68°F	3.68"
August	89°F	67°F	4.22"
September	81°F	61°F	3.24"
October	72°F	49°F	3.40"
November	62°F	39°F	3.14"
December	53°F	32°F	3.25"

Water

How much is enough? Well, one simple physiological fact should convince you to err on the side of excess when deciding how much water to pack: a hiker walking steadily in 90° heat needs to drink approximately 10 quarts of fluid per day. That's 2.5 gallons. A good rule of thumb is to hydrate before your hike, carry (and drink) 6 ounces of water for every mile you plan to hike, and hydrate again after the hike. For most people, the pleasures of hiking make carrying water a relatively minor price to pay to remain safe and healthy.

So pack more water than you anticipate that you'll need, even for short hikes.

If you're tempted to drink "found" water, do so with extreme caution. Many ponds and lakes encountered by hikers are fairly stagnant, and the water tastes terrible. Drinking such water presents inherent risks for thirsty trekkers. The intestinal parasite giardia contaminates many water sources and cause the dreaded illness giardiasis, which can last for weeks after onset. For information, visit the Centers for Disease Control website: **cdc.gov/parasites/giardia.**

In any case, effective purification is essential before you use any water source found along the trail. Boiling water for 2–3 minutes is always a safe measure for camping, but day hikers can consider iodine tablets, approved chemical mixes, filtration units rated for giardia, and ultraviolet filtration. Some of these methods (for example, filtration with an added carbon filter) remove bad tastes typical in stagnant water, while others add their own taste. As a precaution, carry a means of water purification to get you by in a pinch or if you realize you've underestimated your consumption needs.

Clothing

Weather, unexpected trail conditions, fatigue, extended hiking duration, and wrong turns can individually or collectively turn a great outing into a very uncomfortable one at best—and a life-threatening one at worst. Thus, proper attire plays a key role in staying comfortable and, sometimes, in staying alive. Here are some helpful guidelines:

★ Choose silk, wool, or synthetics for maximum comfort—from hats to socks and in between. Cotton is fine if the weather remains dry and stable, but you won't be happy if that material gets wet.

★ Always wear a hat, or at least tuck one into your day pack or hitch it to your belt. Hats offer all-weather sun and wind protection as well as warmth if it turns cold.

★ Be ready to layer up or down as the day progresses and the mercury rises or falls. Today's outdoor wear makes layering easy, with such designs as jackets that convert to vests and zip-off or button-up legs.

★ Wear hiking boots or sturdy hiking sandals with toe protection. Flip-flopping a paved urban greenway is one thing, but never hike a trail in open sandals or casual sneakers. Your bones and arches need support, and your skin needs protection.

★ Pair that footwear with good socks! If you prefer not to sheathe your feet when wearing hiking sandals, tuck some socks into your day pack; you may need them if temperatures plummet or if you hit rocky turf and pebbles begin to irritate your feet. And, in an emergency, if you've lost your gloves, you can adapt the socks into mittens.

★ Don't leave your rain gear at home, even if the day dawns clear and sunny. Tuck into your day pack, or tie around your waist, a jacket that is breathable and either water-resistant or waterproof. Investigate different choices at your local outdoors retailer. If you're a frequent hiker, ideally you'll have more than one rain-gear weight, material, and style in your closet to protect you in all seasons in your regional climate and hiking microclimates.

Essential Gear

Today you can buy outdoor vests that have up to 20 pockets shaped and sized to carry everything from toothpicks to binoculars. Or if you don't aspire to feel like a burro, you can neatly stow all of these items in your day pack or backpack. The following list showcases never-hike-without-them items—in alphabetical order, for easy reference.

★ *Extra clothes:* Rain gear, warm hat, gloves, and change of socks and shirt.

★ *Extra food:* Trail mix, granola bars, or other high-energy foods.

★ *Flashlight or headlamp:* Include extra bulb and batteries.

★ *Insect repellent:* For some areas and seasons, this is extremely vital.

★ *Maps and high-quality compass:* Even if you know the terrain from previous hikes, don't leave home without these tools. And, as previously noted, bring maps in addition to those in this guidebook, and consult your maps prior to the hike. If you are versed in GPS usage, bring that device too, but don't rely on it as your sole navigational tool, as the battery can dwindle or die. And be sure to compare its guidance with that of your maps.

★ *Matches (ideally, windproof) and/or a lighter:* A fire starter is also a good idea.

★ *Pocketknife and/or a multitool:* Never hike without one.

★ *Sunscreen:* Note the expiration date on the tube or bottle.

★ *Water:* As emphasized more than once in this book, bring more than you think you'll drink. Depending on your destination, you may want to bring a water bottle and iodine or filter for purifying water in the wilderness in case you run out.

★ *Whistle:* This little gadget will be your best friend in an emergency.

First-Aid Kit

In addition to the items above, those below may appear overwhelming for a day hike. But any paramedic will tell you that the products listed here, in alphabetical order, are just the basics. The reality of hiking is that you can be out for a week of backpacking and acquire only a mosquito bite—or you can hike for an hour, slip, and suffer a bleeding abrasion or broken bone. Fortunately, these items collapse into a very small space. You may also purchase convenient prepackaged kits at your pharmacy or online.

★ Ace bandages or Spenco joint wraps

★ Antibiotic ointment (Neosporin or the generic equivalent)

★ Athletic tape

★ Band-Aids

★ Benadryl or the generic equivalent, diphenhydramine (in case of allergic reactions)

★ Blister kit (such as Moleskin or Spenco 2nd Skin)

★ Butterfly-closure bandages

★ Epinephrine in a prefilled syringe (for people known to have severe allergic reactions to such things as bee stings; usually available by prescription only)

★ Gauze (one roll and a half dozen 4-x-4-inch pads)

★ Hydrogen peroxide or iodine

★ Ibuprofen or acetaminophen

Note: Consider your intended terrain and the number of hikers in your party before you exclude any article cited in the previous list. A botanical-garden stroll may not inspire you to carry a complete kit, but anything beyond that warrants precaution. When hiking alone, you should always be prepared for a medical need. And if you're part of a twosome or hiking with a group, one or more people in your party should be equipped with first-aid material.

General Safety

The following tips may have the familiar ring of Mom's voice as you take note of them:

★ *Always let someone know* where you'll be hiking and how long you expect to be gone. It's a good idea to give that person a copy of your route, particularly if you're headed into any isolated area. Let that person know when you return.

★ *Always sign in and out of any trail registers provided.* Don't hesitate to comment on the trail condition if space is provided; that's your opportunity to alert others to any problems you encounter.

★ *Never count on a cell phone for your safety.* Reception may be spotty or nonexistent on the trail, even on an urban walk—especially if it's surrounded by towering trees.

★ *Always carry food and water,* even for a short hike. And bring more water than you think you will need. (I cannot say that often enough!)

★ *Ask questions.* State forest and park employees are on hand to help. It's a lot easier to solicit advice before a problem occurs, and it will help you avoid a mishap away from civilization when it's too late to amend an error.

★ *Stay on designated trails.* Even on the most clearly marked trails, there is usually a point where you have to stop and consider in which direction to head. If you become disoriented, don't panic. As soon as you think you may be off-track, stop, assess your current direction, and then retrace your steps to the point where you went astray. Using a map, a compass, and this book, and keeping in mind what you have passed thus far, reorient yourself and trust your judgment on which way to continue. If you become absolutely unsure of how to continue, return to your vehicle the way you came in. Should you become completely lost and have no idea how to return to the trailhead, remaining in place along the trail and waiting for help is most often the best option for adults, and always the best option for children.

★ *Always carry a whistle,* another precaution that cannot be overemphasized. It may be a lifesaver if you do become lost or get hurt.

★ *Be especially careful when crossing streams.* Whether you are fording the stream or crossing on a log, make every step count. If you have any doubt about maintaining your balance on a log, ford the stream instead: use a trekking pole or stout stick for balance and *face upstream as you cross.* If a stream seems too deep to ford, turn back. Whatever is on the other side is not worth risking your life.

★ *Be careful at overlooks.* While these areas may provide spectacular views, they are potentially hazardous. Stay back from the edge of outcrops and be absolutely sure of your footing; a misstep can mean a nasty and possibly fatal fall.

★ *Look up!* Standing dead trees and storm-damaged living ones pose a significant hazard to hikers. These trees may have loose or broken limbs that could fall at any time. Be mindful of this when walking beneath trees, and when choosing a spot to rest or enjoy your snack.

★ *Know hypothermia symptoms.* Shivering and forgetfulness are the two most common indicators of this stealthy killer. Hypothermia can occur at any elevation, even in the summer, especially when the hiker is wearing lightweight cotton clothing. If symptoms present themselves, get to shelter, hot liquids, and dry clothes ASAP.

★ *Likewise, know the symptoms of heat exhaustion (hyperthermia).* Lightheadedness and loss of energy are the first two indicators. If you feel these symptoms, find some shade, drink your water, remove as many layers of clothing as practical, and stay put until you cool down. Marching through heat exhaustion leads to heatstroke—which can be fatal. If you should be sweating and you're not, that's the signature warning sign. Your hike is over at that point—heatstroke is a life-threatening condition that can cause seizures, convulsions, and eventually death. If you or a companion reaches that point, do whatever you can to cool down and seek medical attention immediately.

★ *Most important of all, take along your brain.* A cool, calculating mind is the single most important asset on the trail. Think before you act. Watch your step. Plan ahead. Avoiding accidents before they happen is the best way to ensure a rewarding and relaxing hike.

Watchwords for Flora & Fauna

Hikers should remain aware of the following concerns regarding plant life and wildlife, described in alphabetical order.

BLACK BEARS: Though attacks by black bears are uncommon, they have occurred around Charlotte. The highest concentration of black bears will be found in the western part of the region that is closest to Great Smoky Mountains National Park and also to the east in the Uwharrie National Forest.

The sight or approach of a bear can give anyone a start, but if you encounter a bear while hiking, remain calm and avoid running in any direction. Make loud noises to scare off the bear, and back away slowly. In primitive and remote areas, assume bears are present; in more developed sites, check on the current bear situation prior to hiking. Most encounters are food-related, as bears have an exceptional sense of smell and not particularly discriminating tastes. While this is of greater concern to backpackers and campers, on a day hike you may plan a lunchtime picnic or will munch on an energy bar or other snack from time to time. So remain alert and be particularly cautious about going on a hike or camping after grilling meat. Often the smoke and the smell will get in your hair and on your clothes, and this has been known to be the cause of bear attacks in the past.

BLACK FLIES: Though these insects are certainly pests and maddeningly annoying, the worst a black fly will cause is an itchy welt. They are most active April–June, during the day, and especially before thunderstorms, as well as during the morning and evening hours. Insect repellent has some effect, but the only way to keep out of their swarming midst is to keep moving.

MOSQUITOES: They're certainly a problem in and around Charlotte during the warmer months. During the early spring, the mosquitoes haven't emerged in their full numbers. After the first freeze of the winter, the population is seriously reduced. This makes fall and spring particularly pleasant times to hike and be free of the pestering and itch-inducing buggers. Ward off these pests with insect repellent and/or repellent-impregnated clothing.

Another great way to keep your sanity and avoid being bitten is to wear gloves and a head net. A net draped over a wide-brimmed hat works especially well for keeping all bugs from landing on your face and the back of your neck. In some areas, mosquitoes are known to carry the West Nile virus, so all due caution should be taken to avoid their bites.

POISON IVY, OAK, AND SUMAC: Recognizing and avoiding these plants are the most effective ways to prevent the painful, itchy rashes associated with them. Poison ivy occurs as a vine or ground-cover, 3 leaflets to a leaf; poison oak occurs as a vine or shrub, also with 3 leaflets; and poison sumac flourishes in swampland, each leaf having 7–13 leaflets. Urushiol, the oil in the sap of these plants, is responsible for the rash. Within 14 hours of exposure, raised lines and/or blisters will appear on the affected area, accompanied by a terrible itch.

Try not to scratch if you can—bacteria under your fingernails can cause an infection. Wash and dry the affected area thoroughly, applying a calamine lotion to help dry out the rash. If itching or blistering is severe, seek medical attention. If you do come into contact with one of these plants, remember that oil-contaminated clothes, hiking gear, and pets can easily cause an irritating rash on you or someone else, so wash not only any exposed parts of your body but also any exposed clothes, gear, and pets.

SNAKES: Rattlesnakes, cottonmouths, copperheads, and corals are among the most common venomous snakes in the United States. Their hibernation season is typically October–April. Rattlesnakes like to bask in the sun and won't bite unless threatened.

In the regions described in this book, you will possibly encounter western diamondback rattlesnakes, timber and pygmy rattlers, cottonmouths (water moccasins), and copperheads. However, the snakes you most likely will see while hiking will be nonvenomous species and subspecies. The best rule is to leave all snakes alone, give

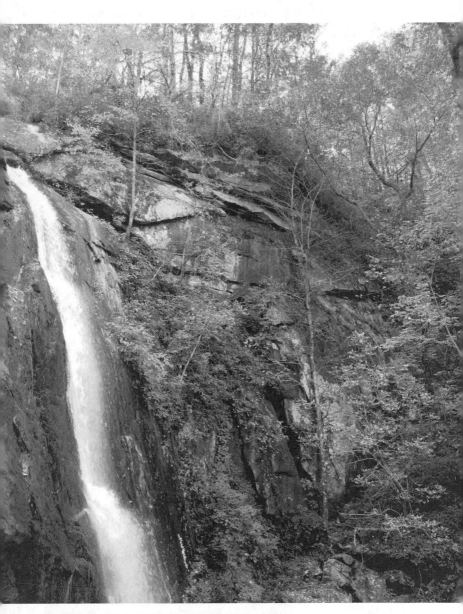

HIGH SHOAL FALLS, SOUTH MOUNTAINS STATE PARK

them a wide berth as you hike past, and make sure any hiking companions (including dogs) do the same.

When hiking, stick to well-used trails, and wear over-the-ankle boots and loose-fitting long pants. Do not step or put your hands beyond your range of detailed visibility, and avoid wandering around in the dark. Step *onto* logs and rocks, never *over* them, and be especially careful when climbing rocks. Always avoid walking through dense brush or willow thickets. Rattlesnakes and copperheads are often found on sunny spots atop rocks, while cottonmouths are likely to be found near lakeshores and along the banks of rivers and creeks.

TICKS: These arachnids are often found on brush and tall grass, where they seem to be waiting to hitch a ride on a warm-blooded passerby. Adult ticks are most active April–May and again October–November. Among the varieties of ticks, the black-legged (deer) tick is the primary carrier of Lyme disease. As a precaution, wear light-colored clothing, which makes it easier for you to spot ticks before they migrate to your skin. At the end of your hike, visually check your hair, back of neck, armpits, and socks. During your posthike shower, take a moment to do a more complete body check. For ticks that are already embedded, removal with tweezers is best. Use disinfectant solution on the wound.

Hunting

Separate rules, regulations, and licenses govern the various hunting types and related seasons. Though there are generally no problems, hikers may wish to forgo their trips during the big-game seasons, when the woods suddenly seem filled with orange and camouflage. The hunting season for most animals in and around Charlotte occurs October–December. The most common places for hikers to encounter hunters are in the Uwharrie National Forest and the Birkhead Wilderness, east of the city.

Regulations

Each state generally has a unique set of rules and regulations that apply to the use of state parks and other public lands. Below you will find many of the most important rules and regulations to know when visiting these areas. Many of these regulations are listed on the rules-and-regulations pages of the North Carolina State Parks and North Carolina Parks and Recreation websites.

★ Pets must be on a leash no longer than 6 feet at all times and must not be left unattended. Campers must confine pets to enclosed vehicles or tents during the park's quiet hours, and pets are not allowed in bathhouses, changing areas, rinsing stations, swimming areas, restrooms, visitor centers, or rental boats. Exceptions are service animals and authorized search-and-rescue dogs.

★ North Carolina state parks are wildlife preserves. The removal, destruction, or injury of any tree, flower, artifact, fern, shrub, rock, or other plant or mineral in any park is prohibited unless you have an approved collection permit for scientific or educational purposes.

★ The hunting, trapping, pursuing, shooting, injuring, killing, or molesting of any bird or animal is prohibited. Feeding or baiting wildlife is prohibited.

★ In parks where boating and fishing are allowed during park hours, such activities are regulated by all applicable North Carolina laws and regulations, including those regarding fishing licenses, boat registration, and safety requirements.

★ For your safety and protection, please stay on designated trails and hiking areas. Also, many rare plants live on thin soils and wet rocks and are vulnerable to damage from climbing, trampling, and scraping.

Camping

★ In North Carolina, it is lawful to camp anywhere in a national forest unless it is otherwise posted. In state parks and national parks, the following are prohibited: alcohol, the possession or use of fireworks, cap pistols, air guns, bows and arrows, slingshots, or lethal missiles of any kind. To possess a handgun within a state or national park, you must carry a concealed-weapon permit; in any case, firearms are prohibited in park offices and visitor centers.

★ As a courtesy to other campers, please observe the campground quiet hours, typically 10 p.m.–7 a.m. In any park or recreation area, sounds that annoy, disturb, or frighten park visitors are prohibited at all times.

★ Camping is allowed in designated areas by permit only. In most cases, campers register with a ranger on-site or at an on-site registration box. Fires are permitted only in designated areas and must be tended at all times. Gathering firewood is generally prohibited but may be allowed in some parks.

Litter

Littering is illegal in North Carolina.

★ To help maintain a clean and safe environment for park visitors and wildlife, place trash in proper containers. Wildlife may mistake plastic bags for food and may become entangled in discarded fishing line or other types of litter.

★ Burying trash is prohibited. Shifting winds and other types of weather may expose trash and endanger wildlife and the environment.

★ State law requires aluminum cans to be placed in recycling containers where available.

Business and Special Activities

Conducting commercial business or activity in any park is prohibited except during events governed by a special-activity permit. Photography or video production for commercial purposes is prohibited unless you have a film permit.

State parks allow for many recreational activities, such as bicycling events, marathons, photo tours, kite-flying contests, club meetings, and so on. However, participants in all such events must acquire a special-activity permit for $35. The permit application is available from the "Forms & Permits" web link at individual park menus or may be obtained from park offices.

Vehicles and Bicycles

★ North Carolina motor-vehicle and traffic laws apply in all state parks. Unlicensed motor vehicles—including golf carts, unregistered motorcycles, snowmobiles, utility vehicles, minibikes, and all-terrain vehicles—are prohibited.

★ Unlicensed drivers may not operate motor vehicles on park roads.

★ Motorized vehicles are permitted only in designated areas and are prohibited on park trails.

★ All vehicles left in the park after posted park hours must be registered.

★ No carts, carriages, or other horse-drawn apparatus are permitted on park trails.

★ In all parks, bicycles are permitted only on those trails or other park areas specifically designated for their use.

★ Bicycle riders under age 16 must wear a helmet.

★ Bicycle passengers who weigh less than 40 pounds or who are less than 40 inches tall must be seated in a separate restraining seat. All other bicycle riders must be seated on saddle seats. Persons unable to maintain an erect, seated position cannot be bicycle passengers.

Trail Etiquette

Always treat trails, wildlife, and fellow hikers with respect. Here are some reminders.

★ Plan ahead in order to be self-sufficient at all times. For example, carry necessary supplies for changes in weather or other conditions. A well-planned trip brings satisfaction to you and to others.

★ Hike on open trails only.

★ In seasons or construction areas where road or trail closures may be a possibility, use the website addresses or phone numbers shown in the "Contacts" line for each of this guidebook's hikes to check conditions prior to heading out for your hike. And do not attempt to circumvent such closures.

★ Avoid trespassing on private land, and obtain all permits and authorization as required. Also, leave gates as you found them or as directed by signage.

★ Be courteous to other hikers, bikers, equestrians, and others you encounter on the trails.

★ Never spook wild animals or pets. An unannounced approach, a sudden movement, or a loud noise startles most critters, and a surprised animal can be dangerous to you, to others, and to itself. Give animals plenty of space.

★ Observe the YIELD signs around the region's trailheads and backcountry. Typically they advise hikers to yield to horses, and bikers to yield to both horses and hikers. Hikers and bikers should yield to any uphill traffic. When encountering mounted riders or horsepackers, hikers can courteously step off the trail, on the downhill side if possible. So that the horse can see and hear you, calmly greet the rider before s/he reaches you, and don't dart behind trees. Also resist the urge to pet a horse unless you're invited to do so.

★ Stay on existing trails, and do not blaze any new ones.

★ Pack out what you pack in, leaving only your footprints. No one likes to see the trash someone else has left behind.

Tips on Enjoying Hiking in Charlotte

It's pretty hard not to enjoy hiking around Charlotte, but a few tips might enhance the experience.

First, check out all of the information listed in this book for the particular trail you consider hiking. Note the contact information and the GPS coordinates of the trailhead. The trail descriptions will help you know what to expect along the trail and help you prepare for such elements as water crossings, fishing opportunities, and views (that is, bring your camera).

Because the trails around Charlotte are fairly spread out, it's always a good idea to see how far a trail may be from your point of origin to avoid driving an hour to a trail when you really just wanted to do a quick day hike. The terrain around Charlotte is also very diverse, and you'll want to consider your own fitness level in making decisions about the level of physical challenge you want to take on.

Take your time on the trail. Hiking presents a great opportunity to relax and think. Hurrying along the trail and becoming too goal-oriented with the process can sometimes take away from the experience.

The main point, though, is to get what you want out of the trail. If you want a physical challenge—to run the trails, time yourself, and attempt to set new records—do it. If you want to take a whole day to hike a few miles, sitting and picnicking and watching the clouds roll by, then you should set aside a day to do just that. Whatever you do, make sure to hike the trail in your own way and make it *your* experience.

Just as important as it is to never live anyone else's life, you should never hike anyone else's trail.

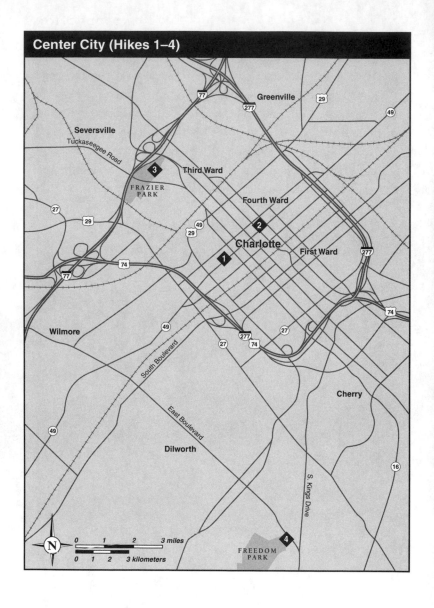

Center City (Hikes 1–4)

77

277

Greenville 29

49

Seversville

Tuckaseegee Road

Third Ward

3

FRAZIER PARK

Fourth Ward

27

29

49

29

2

Charlotte

First Ward

277

74

77

74

49

Wilmore

49

South Boulevard

277

27

74

27

74

East Boulevard

Cherry

49

Dilworth

S. Kings Drive

16

N

0   1   2   3 miles

0   1   2   3 kilometers

FREEDOM PARK

4

Center City

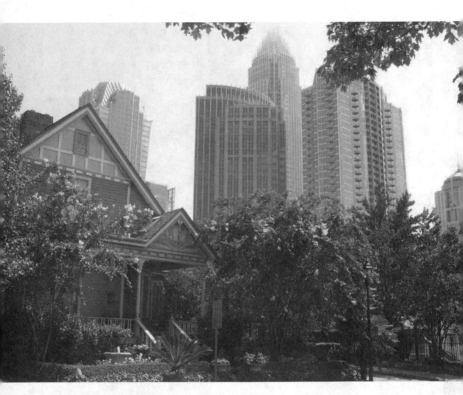

EXPLORE ONE OF CHARLOTTE'S EARLIEST PROSPEROUS NEIGHBORHOODS ON A WALK THROUGH THE FOURTH WARD.

Downtown–Uptown Walk

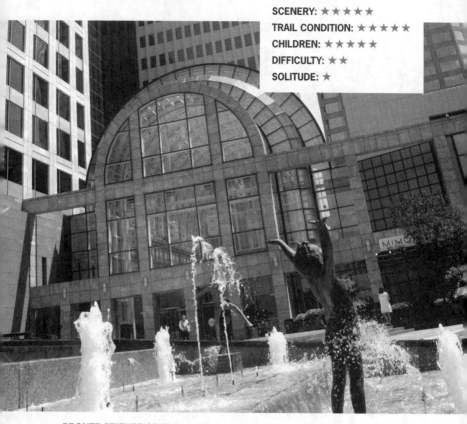

SCENERY: ★ ★ ★ ★ ★
TRAIL CONDITION: ★ ★ ★ ★ ★
CHILDREN: ★ ★ ★ ★ ★
DIFFICULTY: ★ ★
SOLITUDE: ★

BRONZE STATUES OF CHILDREN PLAYING IN A FOUNTAIN ADD A TOUCH OF PLAYFULNESS TO CHARLOTTE'S CITY CENTER.

GPS COORDINATES: Visitor Info Center: N35° 13.494' W80° 50.798'

DISTANCE & CONFIGURATION: 3.0-mile loop

HIKING TIME: 3 hours

HIGHLIGHTS: Uptown Charlotte and The Green park

ELEVATION: Negligible—743'–762'

ACCESS: 24/7 but not recommended after dark due to crime and poor lighting in some areas

MAPS: At Charlotte Visitor Info Center, the Charlotte Convention Center, or **charlottesgotalot.com**

FACILITIES: Water fountains at The Green (a park)

WHEELCHAIR ACCESS: Yes, but navigation may be difficult on some sidewalks.

COMMENTS: Avoid morning and evening rush hours, as this route passes through a congested area of Uptown Charlotte and requires crossing many roads with frequent traffic.

CONTACTS: Charlotte Visitor Info Center (Center City location): (704) 331-2700; **charlottesgotalot.com**

Overview

This route explores the heart of Downtown and Uptown Charlotte, taking you past some of the most visited attractions that really capture the spirit and character of the city. Nestled among impressive examples of urban development and towering buildings are historic sites, art displays, and entertainment venues. The loop route begins at the Visitor Info Center, Center City location (other branches are at the airport and at the Levine Museum of the New South, not near this route), where you can pick up a free illustrated city map. From there you'll meander some dozen blocks and cross through a wonderful park as you loop back to the Visitor Info Center. This trail is a treat for children old enough to walk 3 miles, as there are lots of interesting sites and adventures for them along this route. In fact, you should spend a few minutes at the Visitor Info Center to decide on any attractions that may capture your attention along the way— and plan your time accordingly.

Route Details

Start at the Visitor Info Center (noted by a circular red sign with a white lowercase *i* for "information") on South Tryon Street between West Third Street and West Martin Luther King Jr. (MLK Jr.) Boulevard. Follow Tryon north toward Third Street. On the way to Third Street, look to your right at the artfully crafted bronze statues of children playing and splashing in the fountain waters.

Continue north on Tryon and pass Ruth's Chris Steak House on your left. Trolleys run along Tryon Street, so feel free to hop aboard

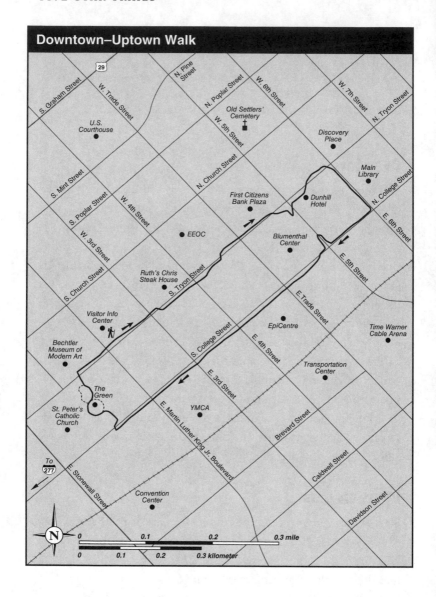

Downtown–Uptown Walk

if you'd like a lift to a particular location along the Tryon Street route of this walk. Continue on Tryon and cross Fourth Street, passing the decorative and architecturally interesting Tryon Plaza on your right and First Citizens Bank Plaza on your left, where you are likely to see locals playing cards and chess games around the tables in front of the waterfall on the side of the building.

Continue to the Trade Street junction, where South Tryon becomes North Tryon and West Trade becomes East Trade. This is the official center of the city. The large and impressive statues on each corner here represent Charlotte's commerce, transportation, industry, and future. Also, the first courthouse was built at this confluence and, according to some historians, the Mecklenburg Declaration of Independence was read here, in 1775, during the American Revolution. With that declaration, the area's colonists announced their desire to separate from England—prior to the 1776 Declaration of Independence.

Cross Trade Street and continue north on Tryon. A Starbucks will be on your left, which will appeal to you if you are interested in stopping for a coffee. Cross East Fifth Street, walking toward The Capital Grille, the Wooden Vine Wine Bar and Bistro, and the historic Dunhill Hotel on your left. On the corner of Sixth and Tryon is the Discovery Place, a hands-on science museum for kids. It is very well done, with a really neat rainforest exhibit, aquarium, and, best of all, an IMAX theater. But if you want to save that for another time and continue the walk, turn right (southeast) onto East Sixth Street, where you'll see the large Charlotte Mecklenburg Library on your left, and walk one block to North College Street, where Fuel Pizza sits on the corner. To your left you have a sharp view of Transamerica Square's gold dome peeking through the trees.

At College Street, turn right (southwest). In a few strides, you'll see The Trade Center on your left. The complex encompasses a variety of shops and restaurants that cater to the business-class workers in this area. Of note is Mert's Heart and Soul restaurant, in case you're pining for some of Mert's fried green tomatoes or, as his menu declares, his Famous Salmon Cakes to sustain you on your foray.

Cross East Fifth Street, with the impressive dome of the Time Warner Cable Arena visible to the left. The arena hosts various music concerts and performance acts, is home to the National Basketball Association's Charlotte Bobcats, and was the scene of the 2012 Democratic National Convention.

At the intersection of Trade and College streets—where North College becomes South College—you will see the popular Omni Hotel and the Charlotte EpiCentre complex. EpiCentre hosts a movie theater, Moe's Southwest Grill, a CVS, and several bagel shops, among other chain restaurant and retail stores. Turn left (southwest) onto South College. The Bank of America Corporate Tower, the largest building in Charlotte, rises above the Omni Hotel to your right.

Continue southward on College and cross East Fourth Street, with Charlotte Plaza on your left, then East Third Street, with the Hilton Hotel to your left. Keep walking southwest to cross MLK Jr. Boulevard, and then continue down South College until you reach the stair entrance to The Green, a 1.5-acre park, on your right. This is definitely Uptown Charlotte's best park, wonderfully accented with colorful literary-themed statues covered in mosaic tiles. Children find it particularly delightful.

Turn right (northwest) and walk through the park's center to South Tryon Street, passing the fantastic and way-larger-than-life goldfish fountain on the left. You can also dine outdoors or inside at one of the restaurants that line The Green.

Once you reach South Tryon Street, turn right (northeast) along Tryon and cross MLK Jr. Boulevard again, where you arrive directly across the street from the Visitor Info Center where you started. At this point, you'll likely want to sample its open-air courtyard with a number of tables and chairs, where you can have a rest at the end of your Charlotte city walk.

Nearby Attractions

There is so much near Charlotte's city center. Of note and not already covered in the route is the Bank of America Stadium, home to the Charlotte Panthers of the National Football League. Also nearby is Charlotte's historic Fourth Ward district (see next profile), where you can explore some of the city's best-preserved historic homes. South of this route on MLK Jr. Boulevard is the NASCAR Hall of Fame, which is definitely worth checking out for all you checkered-flag fans. Latta Plantation (see page 60) is about 1 mile south of Uptown near the Carolinas Medical Center and can be accessed by going south on South Caldwell Street to South Boulevard from the city center.

Directions

From I-77 North, take Exit 10 to West Trade Street and turn right (east) onto Trade Street. From I-77 South, take Exit 10B to West Trade Street and turn right (east) onto West Trade Street. As you drive into the Uptown area, street-corner green and orange signs will direct you to the Visitor Info Center so that you can get close and then find parking nearby.

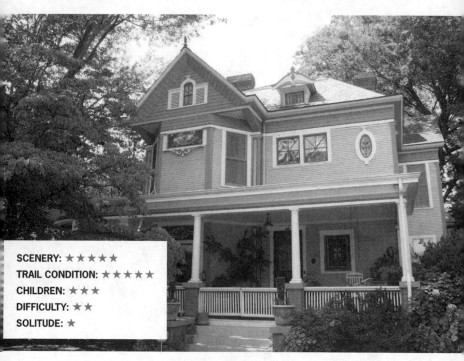

SCENERY: ★ ★ ★ ★ ★
TRAIL CONDITION: ★ ★ ★ ★ ★
CHILDREN: ★ ★ ★
DIFFICULTY: ★ ★
SOLITUDE: ★

GRAND OLD HOMES LINE THE PICTURESQUE STREETS OF CHARLOTTE'S FOURTH WARD.

GPS TRAILHEAD COORDINATES: West Fifth and North Tryon streets: N35° 13.693'
W80° 50.510'

DISTANCE & CONFIGURATION: 2.6-mile figure eight

HIKING TIME: 3 hours

HIGHLIGHTS: Historic homes, Uptown Charlotte, Old Settlers' Cemetery, Fourth Ward Park, and Booth Gardens

ELEVATION: 752' at the trailhead to 718' at lowest point

ACCESS: 24/7 but not recommended after dark due to crime and poor lighting in some areas

MAPS: At Charlotte Visitor Info Center or **charlottesgotalot.com** (click on "Maps")

FACILITIES: Water fountains at Fourth Ward Park

WHEELCHAIR ACCESS: Yes, but navigation may be difficult on some sidewalks.

COMMENTS: Avoid morning and evening rush hours; this route passes through a congested area of Uptown and will require crossing many roads with frequent traffic.

CONTACTS: Friends of Fourth Ward: **fofw.org**

Overview

This walk explores the historic heart of Charlotte's Uptown city center. In the 1800s, four political divisions made up the city's geographic footprint, and the prosperous neighborhood in the northwest section of the city became the Fourth Ward. Over time, the neighborhood fell into disrepair and remained that way until a newly minted 1970s neighborhood association sought to restore the area's homes and business properties. Today, this district embraces some of the city's finest examples of residential architecture by any standards, and on this route you will travel among the Fourth Ward's best blocks of homes, parks, and attractions. Consider making this walk during the holiday season, when many of the historic homes are open to the public for touring, or in the spring and fall when the weather is most pleasant.

Route Details

The route begins on the corner of West Fifth and North Tryon streets. You will be near the Blumenthal Performing Arts Center, and you can't miss seeing The Capital Grille. Most locals can direct you toward that business district fine-dining restaurant, should you need reassurance that you're moving in the right direction to the starting point.

The only public water fountains along this route are in Fourth Ward Park, so you may want to stop in at one of the area's shops and pick up a snack or drink before you stride into the residential district that lies beyond.

From the West Fifth–North Tryon intersection, head northwest on Fifth Street, passing Qboda Mexican Grill on your left. Walk one block to North Church Street, with Basil Thai restaurant on the right and Molly MacPherson's Scottish Pub & Grill on your left. On the northwest corner of Church and Fifth, you will see the Old Settlers'

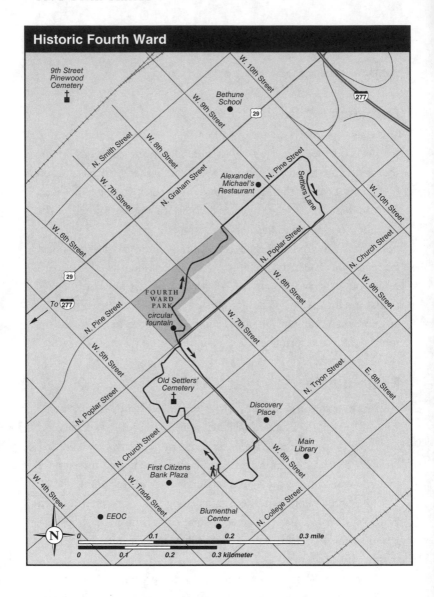

Historic Fourth Ward

Cemetery, bordered by a waist-high stone wall. Cross Church Street and walk up the six stone steps on the cemetery's Fifth Street side that lead to the clay-brick path and the entrance to Settlers'. On the opposite side of Fifth Street, you'll see the First Presbyterian Church, built in 1857. The Victorian Gothic–style church has a noteworthy Tiffany window on the third floor, Church Street side.

Turning your attention back to the cemetery, follow the clay-brick path and walk the length of Charlotte's oldest cemetery along Fifth Street. The first grave here is dated 1776. At the end of the Fifth Street boundary, turn right (northeast) to continue on the clay-brick path toward the redbrick apartment buildings straight ahead. Exit the cemetery onto Poplar Street, and walk less than a block toward Fourth Ward Park's entrance at the corner of North Poplar and West Sixth streets. Cross Sixth Street straight ahead (northeast) and then turn left (northwest), crossing Poplar Street. Walk past the circular fountain that defines the entrance to Fourth Ward Park, and follow the redbrick-paved path through the center of the park. Mostly modern apartment and condo developments surround the park; along the path you pass several benches, water fountains, and a playground, and you will come to the nicely landscaped Booth Gardens. Continue on to the Eighth Street exit of the park and turn left (northwest) toward the park's Pine Street boundary.

Here you enter the core of the Fourth Ward residential district and its streets lined with quintessential Victorian and Southern architectural–style homes. Many of them are truly magnificent. Follow along Eighth Street and then turn right (northeast) onto North Pine Street, where a fountain bubbles in the courtyard to your left and a hard-to-miss, very large, and very pink house stands on the corner to your right. Follow the brick sidewalk along Pine toward West Ninth Street. At the end of the block on your left is the highly recommended Alexander Michael's Restaurant, serving a variety of tasty and reasonably priced dishes from a pretty international menu. This is a great spot to stop for lunch. They also have a nice selection of beers and microbrews and an appreciable wine list.

Cross West Ninth Street and continue on North Pine, around the curve where Pine turns into Settlers Lane and is lined with newer upscale apartments and town homes. You will come to North Poplar Street, where you turn right (southwest) and follow Poplar down to West Seventh Street. From this perspective, you can enjoy great views of the Uptown buildings rising behind the beautifully restored historic homes that line this street.

Cross West Seventh Street and continue southwest on North Poplar toward West Sixth Street. Turn left (southeast) on West Sixth Street, walking one block southeast toward Church Street and then another block southeast toward North Tryon Street. Once you reach North Tryon, turn right (southwest) and continue on to the corner of West Fifth and North Tryon. You've come back to the beginning of your walk, in front of The Capital Grille.

Nearby Attractions

The Fourth Ward is an easy walk to everything in Charlotte's city center, a busy business and tourism district. An exceptional number of attractions, restaurants, and hotels beckon locals and visitors alike. The Bank of America Stadium is about 0.25 mile southwest of the Fourth Ward. Some notable hotels in the area are the Omni, Marriott, Aloft, Hilton Garden Inn, and the historic Dunhill. Aside from Alexander Michael's, which you saw at the corner of North Pine and West Ninth streets, other notable restaurants in the area are Mert's Heart and Soul and the Dandelion Market.

Directions

This route is almost smack-dab in the center of Uptown Charlotte, which begins at the intersection of North and South Tryon streets and East and West Trade streets. (South of this intersection is Downtown Charlotte.) From I-77 North, take Exit 10 to West Trade Street and turn right (east) onto West Trade Street. From I-77 South, take Exit 10B to West Trade Street and turn right (east) onto West Trade Street.

3 # Irwin Creek and Stewart Creek Greenway

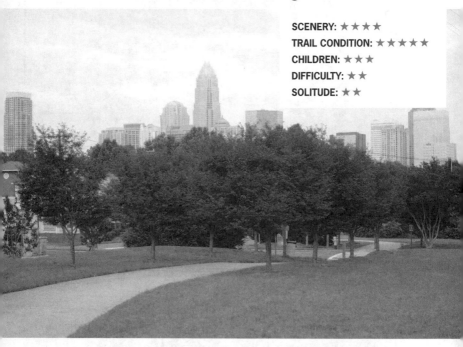

SCENERY: ★ ★ ★ ★
TRAIL CONDITION: ★ ★ ★ ★ ★
CHILDREN: ★ ★ ★
DIFFICULTY: ★ ★
SOLITUDE: ★ ★

THE CHARLOTTE SKYLINE PEEKS ABOVE THE TREES THAT LINE THE GREENWAY.

GPS TRAILHEAD COORDINATES: Bridge trailhead: N35° 14.058' W80° 51.334'

DISTANCE & CONFIGURATION: 2.5-mile out-and-back

HIKING TIME: 2 hours

HIGHLIGHTS: Frazier Park, dog park, Irwin Creek, Seversville Park, and historic Wesley Heights neighborhood

ELEVATION: 634' at the trailhead to 679'

ACCESS: 24/7 but not recommended after dark due to poor lighting in the area

MAPS: At Charlotte Visitor Info Center or **parkandrec.com**

FACILITIES: Restrooms and water fountains

WHEELCHAIR ACCESS: Only on concrete paths throughout Frazier Park

COMMENTS: Trail is shared with bikers, runners, inline skaters, and skateboarders, and leashed dogs are allowed.

CONTACTS: (704) 432-1570; **parkandrec.com**

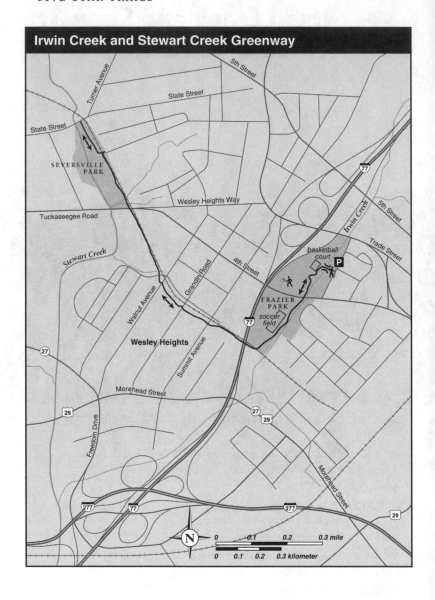

Irwin Creek and Stewart Creek Greenway

Overview

This trail is part of Charlotte's impressive greenway system. To date, the Charlotte area has 14 greenways containing more than 30 miles of trails, making it one of the best greenway systems in the country. This route begins at Frazier Park in Charlotte's Uptown city-center area. At Frazier Park, the trail passes basketball courts, a dog park, soccer field, tennis courts, and a playground before traveling through the historic Wesley Heights neighborhood and reaching Seversville Park for the turnaround point. Make sure to bring a basketball, soccer ball, or tennis balls and racquets if you're interested in mixing these activities into your walk. One portion of the trail follows an old railroad bed and through a forested area of Uptown Charlotte. The proximity of the trail to Johnson & Wales University (renowned for its culinary programs) and the nearby restaurant and business plaza make the trail a popular excursion while visiting Charlotte's city center.

Route Details

The trail begins in front of the wooden bridge with metal handrails. Walk toward the basketball court on the opposite side of the bridge and take a left (southwest). Continue on the 6-foot-wide concrete path and pass the tennis courts and dog park on the right side. Dogs are allowed on the trail as long as they are kept on a 6-foot (or shorter) leash, and friendly canines are welcome to roam free in the dog park, defined by the chain-link fence.

Follow the arrows painted onto the path and walk under the artistic Fourth Street overpass. Its mural of flowers exemplifies the greenway's public art displays. To your right you will note a soccer field and a small playground. The trees that border the soccer field offer a shady spot for watching a local soccer match or to rest and enjoy a picnic. Several water fountains avail themselves along this portion of the trail around the soccer field and playground areas.

The path follows alongside Irwin Creek to the right and enters into the beginning of the historic Wesley Heights neighborhood also on the right. Pass the disc-golf basket on the right, or stop and practice a few throws and then continue along the creek. The trail circles around the soccer field and then arcs over train tracks before going under the overpass for I-77. Cross Summit Avenue and continue to follow the signs toward the Irwin Belk Complex, an athletics facility on the campus of Johnson C. Smith University. This section of the greenway is very pleasant and lined with sycamore trees that provide welcome shade in the hotter spring and summer months. Continue on the paved path, crossing Grandin Road and Walnut Avenue. The fieldstone column-type markers outfitted with metal plaques denote the street names and will ease your navigation, and the concrete path on this section is very well defined. It's hard to get lost on this greenway.

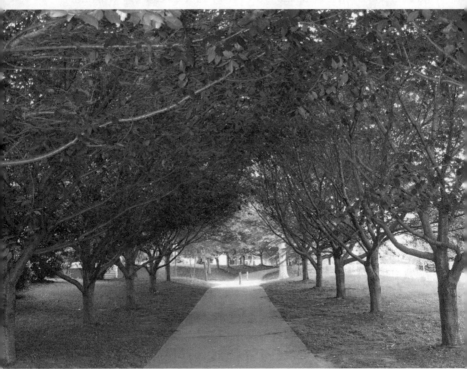

THE TREE-LINED PATH OFFERS A SHADY RESPITE FROM THE SPRING AND SUMMER HEAT.

Turn right on the gravel path that follows along the train tracks. The trail enters into a forested area that is very fragrant in the spring and summer with the scents of wildflowers and honeysuckle. Many spur trails connect to neighborhoods along this forested section. Stay straight on the main gravel path that follows the abandoned railroad bed. Go under the overpass at the end of the forested section, and enter Seversville Park. Stay straight on the gravel trail. To the right are spacious picnic pavilions and a large playground. Benches throughout the park and plentiful shady spots beneath the park's trees offer nice resting spots. The trail ends where you turn around and head back to your starting point, at the wooden bridge in Frazier Park.

Nearby Attractions

This is a popular recreation and running spot for the locals living and working in the new urban residential area of Gateway Village. Around Gateway and along Trade Street, you'll find several plazas with a variety of good restaurants and bars where you can stop in for a bite to eat or grab a drink. If it's summertime and you're ready to cool off after a day in the sweltering heat, you can head to Ray's Splash Planet, a water park within walking distance of Frazier Park. Bank of America Stadium is less than a mile southeast from the greenway, and farther to the east is the heart of Charlotte's Uptown city center, packed with restaurants, bars, entertainment, attractions, and fine hotels, including the four-star Omni.

Directions

From Charlotte's city center, take I-277 North and merge onto I-77 North at Exit 1C toward Statesville. Take the Trade Street exit at Exit 10 toward Fifth Street. Turn left onto West Trade Street and then continue to Frazier Park at 1201 West Trade Street on the left. To hike the Irwin Creek Greenway, park along South Sycamore Street or at the Frazier Park car lot.

Little Sugar Creek Greenway

SCENERY: ★ ★ ★ ★
TRAIL CONDITION: ★ ★ ★ ★ ★
CHILDREN: ★ ★ ★
DIFFICULTY: ★ ★
SOLITUDE: ★

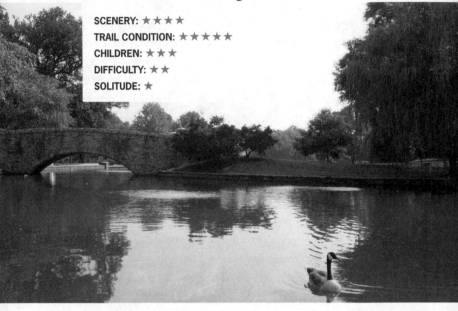

LITTLE SUGAR CREEK GREENWAY FOLLOWS ALONGSIDE A POND IN FREEDOM PARK.

GPS TRAILHEAD COORDINATES: N35° 11.750' W80° 50.301'

DISTANCE & CONFIGURATION: 4.4-mile out-and-back

HIKING TIME: 3 hours

HIGHLIGHTS: Freedom Park, sculptures, and Little Sugar Creek

ELEVATION: 612' at the trailhead to 624'

ACCESS: 24/7

MAPS: At Charlotte Visitor Info Center or **parkandrec.com**

FACILITIES: Restrooms, water fountains, lake, amphitheater, and picnic shelters

WHEELCHAIR ACCESS: Freedom Park and restrooms are accessible.

COMMENTS: The rail is shared with bikers, runners, inline skaters, and skateboarders, and leashed dogs are allowed.

CONTACTS: (704) 432-1570; **parkandrec.com**

Overview

This 2.2-mile section of the Little Sugar Creek Greenway connects the Carolinas Medical Center with the recreation activities of Freedom Park and two other smaller parks to the south. This route is part of a larger linear-park greenway project throughout Charlotte that aims to reduce flooding, clean the waterways, and provide more green space and outdoor activities to residents. To date there are 14 greenways in the Charlotte area that contain more than 30 miles of trails, making it one of the best greenway systems in the country.

Route Details

This route, a section of the Little Sugar Creek Greenway, begins at the northern end of Freedom Park, near the Carolinas Medical Center on Blythe Boulevard. Freedom Park is open to hikers, runners, inline skaters, skateboarders, and bikers. You may park along the road entrance to Freedom Park and also in front of the tennis courts in the lot on Maryland Avenue.

From the parking lot in front of the tennis courts, concrete stairs lead up to a concrete pad bordered by wooden benches. On the far side of the concrete pad, another set of stairs leads down to a 4-foot-wide concrete path that runs behind the tennis courts and alongside Little Sugar Creek. Follow the path past the sports complex on the right with baseball, basketball, and softball fields. Note how the greenway is integrated into neighborhoods and individual residences; along this section you will also notice several smaller footpaths that lead out of the park into neighborhoods and the backyards of private properties. Magnolia, oak, and pine trees border the trail, with its understory of lantana and other wildflowers.

Once you reach the bridge spanning Little Sugar Creek, turn right (northwest) and continue walking west in Freedom Park. After 400 feet, you will reach a playground. Turn left to access a stone bridge that crosses the small stream. You will come to a number of notables: a beautiful pond bordered by willow trees, several fountains,

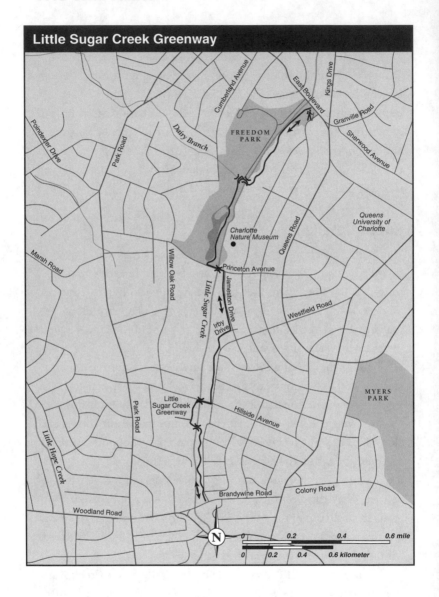

Little Sugar Creek Greenway

an expansive lawn, a playground, picnic shelters, restrooms, and an amphitheater. Masterfully crafted stone bridges accent the charm of the large pond, where families of ducks and geese wade and play. Follow the trail past the picnic pavilions and continue along the shore of the Freedom Park pond.

For the next 0.4 mile, the trail continues pleasantly along the pond shore, passing a cable suspension bridge that leads left to the Charlotte Nature Museum. Water fountains appear at regular intervals in Freedom Park and are a welcome sight on a hot summer day. Continue walking southwest until you reach the edge of Freedom Park. Here you will cross Princeton Avenue and continue on Jameston Drive, where the greenway travels through a quiet neighborhood. After 0.3 mile, take a right (southwest) onto Irby Drive and then take your next right (south) onto Westfield Road. The neighborhood residents here have clearly embraced the greenway, and along the route you are likely to spot several dog bowls filled with water and small handcrafted signs welcoming dogs to a refreshing drink. (Unfortunately, there were no charming signs offering cheeseburgers to hungry guidebook writers.)

After 0.2 mile, cross Hillside Avenue and then turn right (west). Follow Hillside for just 300 feet and then cross a bridge that spans over Little Sugar Creek. At the other side of the small bridge, turn left (south) onto the greenway that runs alongside Little Sugar Creek once again. Follow the trail for 0.4 mile, crossing another metal bridge over Little Sugar Creek. Along this section, you will enjoy a number of wildlife sculptures and other works depicting humans at play. Here also, several flat rock outcrops overhang the creek and make for a nice resting or picnic stop.

Continue along Westfield Road until you reach the end of the Little Sugar Creek Greenway. Plum trees surround a redbrick paved park with bike racks and benches. Before turning around to head back to your starting point, enjoy the shade of a single sycamore tree in the center of the well-designed area.

Nearby Attractions

Adjacent to Freedom Park, the Charlotte Nature Museum houses many exhibits and live animals and has a beautiful garden to explore. Admission is $6 per person (adults and children). Many restaurants and pubs near the greenway, particularly along East Boulevard, can satisfy your appetite after a day on the trail.

Directions

From Downtown Charlotte, head southwest on South Tryon Street toward West Fourth Street. After 0.6 mile, turn left onto East Morehead Street. Drive 1.1 miles and then turn right onto Kenilworth Avenue. Drive 0.5 mile and turn left onto East Boulevard. Drive 0.5 mile, and the entrance to Freedom Park will be on the right. The tennis court's parking-lot entrance is directly after the road entrance to Freedom Park.

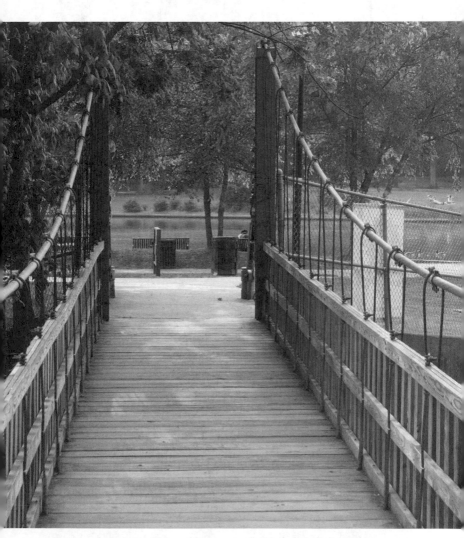

A CABLE SUSPENSION BRIDGE LEADS TO THE CHARLOTTE NATURE MUSEUM.

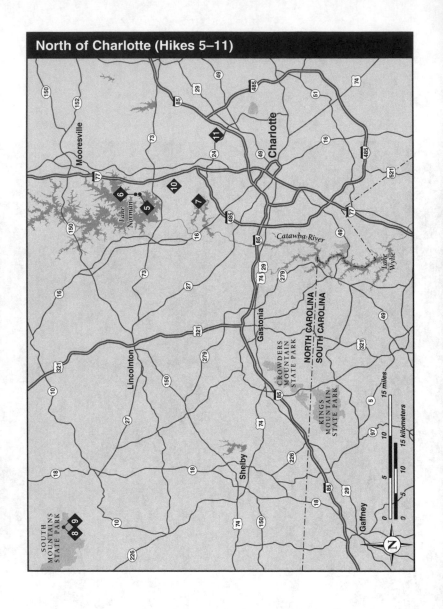

North of Charlotte (Hikes 5–11)

North of Charlotte

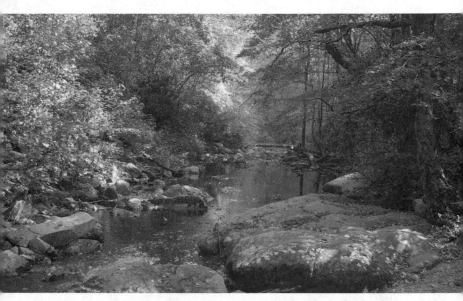

WALKING THE TRAILS OF SOUTH MOUNTAINS STATE PARK MAKES YOU FEEL AS
IF YOU'RE HIKING IN THE HEART OF THE SOUTHERN APPALACHIANS.

5

Jetton Park: Loop 1

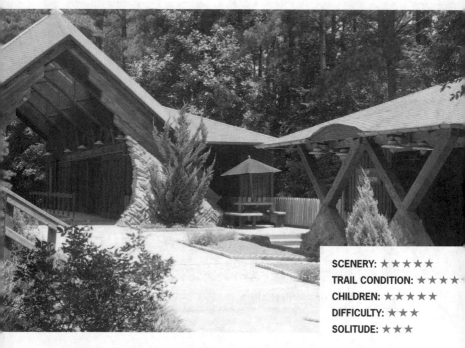

SCENERY: ★ ★ ★ ★ ★
TRAIL CONDITION: ★ ★ ★ ★
CHILDREN: ★ ★ ★ ★ ★
DIFFICULTY: ★ ★ ★
SOLITUDE: ★ ★ ★

JETTON PARK TRAILS ARE POPULAR WITH HIKERS, RUNNERS, AND BIKERS.

GPS TRAILHEAD COORDINATES: Park Office: N35° 28.106' W80° 54.043'

DISTANCE & CONFIGURATION: 0.9-mile loop

HIKING TIME: 1.5 hours

HIGHLIGHTS: Lake Norman, pavilion, gardens, and beach

ELEVATION: 770' at the trailhead to 788'

ACCESS: Daily, 9 a.m.–9 p.m.; March–October: Saturday–Sunday and holidays, $3 per vehicle (county resident) or $5 per vehicle (non–county resident)

MAPS: At Charlotte Visitor Info Center, kiosks at the trailhead and around the park, and **parkandrec.com**

FACILITIES: Restrooms, visitor center, picnic pavilions, boat ramp, and water fountains

WHEELCHAIR ACCESS: Yes, for restrooms, visitor center, picnic pavilions, and paved portions of trails

COMMENTS: Trail is shared with bikers, runners, and inline skaters, and dogs are allowed on leashes 6 feet (or shorter) in length.

CONTACTS: (704) 432-7600 or (704) 336-8869; **parkandrec.com** (search for "Jetton Park")

Overview

Located about 25 minutes north of Charlotte's city center, the 105-acre Jetton Park has more than 4 miles of trails to explore. This hike starts at the park's visitor center, on the shore of Lake Norman, and follows a section of the larger 1.5-mile loop trail onto smaller trails that lead into the center of the park, where formal gardens and a gazebo nestle in a mature pine-and-hardwood forest. The trail meanders through the gardens before rejoining the main trail on the lakeshore, then leads to a spacious sunning beach and picnic area before returning to the visitor center and the trailhead.

Route Details

The walking trail begins at the park office. Follow the paved path from the parking lot toward the lake. Turn left (east) at the concrete path in front of the restrooms. It continues through an A-frame building faced with artfully crafted stonework and topped with a skylight. Pass through the A-frame structure and exit onto the paved path that leads into the mature pine and hardwood forest. Blue and white mile markers line the trail, so you can keep track of how far you've walked.

Throughout this park you will find numerous picnic pavilions. Some are open on a first-come, first-serve basis, while others must be reserved in advance. Signs on the front of each picnic pavilion will tell you whether you are able to use them spontaneously. Most of them offer views of the lake and are equipped with barbecue grills. After following the asphalt trail for approximately 0.1 mile, turn left (west) toward the gazebo. Cross the road and follow the gravel-and-dirt path on the other side. To the left you see the park's commemorative plaque. Stay straight on the trail to continue through Jetton's gardens.

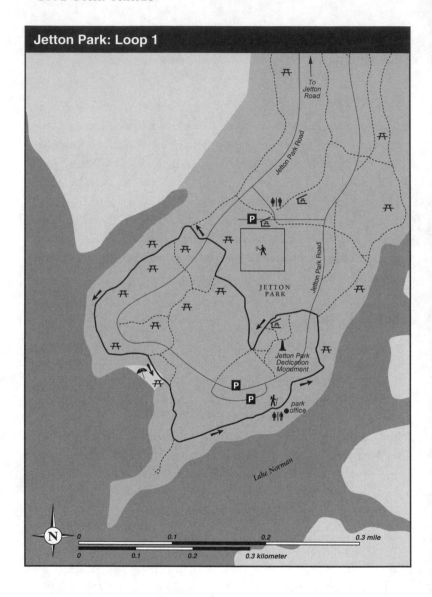

Jetton Park: Loop 1

A wonderful variety of trees and flowers and a nice display of azaleas fill the garden with color throughout the spring and summer. The trail passes a small gazebo in the center of the garden, which is a nice place to sit and take in the beautiful landscape, enjoying the sound of birds chirping and couples volleying on the nearby tennis courts in the distance. Stay straight on the gravel trail and continue to where the trail splits in four directions. Turn right (north) and follow a 5-foot-wide gravel path through the forest.

Turn right (northeast) where the trail curves toward the northwest and then crosses a paved road. Continue on the gravel path and turn left (southwest) where the path becomes asphalt and begins to run beside a northwest arm of Lake Norman. After another 0.1 mile, you reach the sunning beach on your right. No swimming is allowed at the beach, but it's still a great spot for sunbathing and relaxing, with a nice view of Lake Norman. Behind the beach are several picnic tables in a grove of tall pines.

Continue on the paved trail, which veers slightly to the right to an observation area with more views of Lake Norman. Stay straight on the trail to continue back to the visitor center, restrooms, trailhead, and parking lot where your journey began.

Nearby Attractions

The park is encircled on three sides by Lake Norman, and a boat ramp provides access to the lake activities. About 0.5 mile to the west is the Peninsula Golf Club—handy if you are in the mood to hit the links. The 43-acre Ramsey Creek Park, about a mile to the south down West Catawba Road, features more nature trails, another boat ramp, and Lake Norman access, as well as a 3-acre dog park. Concessions and lodging are available in the nearby town of Davidson, about 3 miles to the northeast.

Directions

From the Charlotte city center, take I-277 South to I-77 North at Exit 1C toward Statesville. Follow I-77 for 18.6 miles, and then take Exit 28 to US 21 South toward Lake Norman, and follow it for 0.2 mile. Turn left onto East Catawba Avenue and follow it for 1.2 miles. Turn right onto Jetton Road and follow it for 0.4 mile, and then turn into Jetton Park on your left. Drive into Jetton Park and pass the entrance gate and booth. Here you enter onto a one-way road. Drive past the playground and parking area on your left, and continue until you reach the visitor center, picnic pavilion, and parking lot on your right. Park here and walk toward the visitor center.

6

Jetton Park: Loop 2

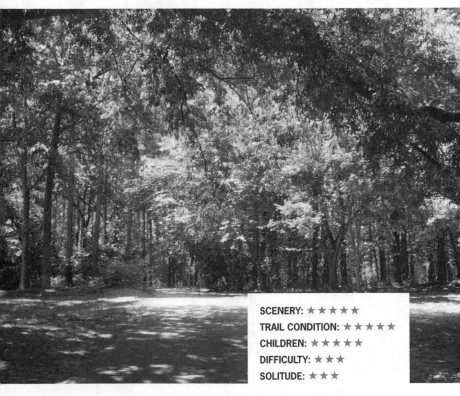

SCENERY: ★ ★ ★ ★ ★
TRAIL CONDITION: ★ ★ ★ ★ ★
CHILDREN: ★ ★ ★ ★ ★
DIFFICULTY: ★ ★
SOLITUDE: ★ ★ ★

A SHADED SECTION OF THE PAVED TRAIL THROUGH JETTON PARK PASSES THROUGH A PINE-AND-HARDWOOD FOREST.

GPS TRAILHEAD COORDINATES: N35° 28.453' W80° 54.017'

DISTANCE & CONFIGURATION: 1.4-mile loop

HIKING TIME: 2 hours

HIGHLIGHTS: Lake Norman, pavilion, and beach

ELEVATION: 852' at the trailhead to 742' at the lowest point

ACCESS: Daily, 9 a.m.–9 p.m.; March–October: Saturday–Sunday and holidays, $3 per vehicle (county resident) or $5 per vehicle (non–county resident)

MAPS: At Charlotte Visitor Info Center, kiosks at the trailhead and around the park, and **parkandrec.com**

FACILITIES: Restrooms, visitor center, picnic pavilions, boat ramp, and water fountains

Jetton Park: Loop 2

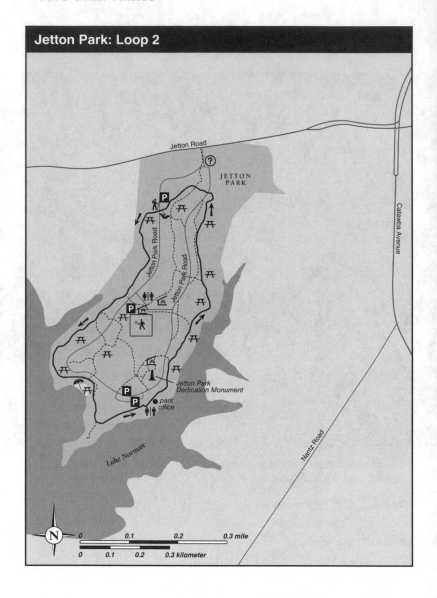

WHEELCHAIR ACCESS: Yes, for restrooms, visitor center, picnic pavilions, and paved portions of trails

COMMENTS: Trail is shared with bikers, runners, and inline skaters, and dogs are allowed on leashes 6 feet (or shorter) in length.

CONTACTS: (704) 432-7600 or (704) 336-8869; **parkandrec.com** (search for "Jetton Park")

Overview

This route follows a biking and running path that runs along the outer edge of 105-acre Jetton Park, about 25 minutes north of Charlotte's city center. The trail begins at a playground near the entrance of the park and follows the path through a mature pine and hardwood forest before reaching the shore of Lake Norman. Along the lakeshore, many picnic pavilions equipped with barbecue grills offer wonderful views of the lake. The path also leads to a sunning beach before it returns to the playground and the trailhead.

Route Details

Proceed to the trailhead to the west behind the parking lot. The paved trail runs through a forest of mature pine and hardwood trees. Picnic tables dot the edge of the trail. Most of them are shaded and offer

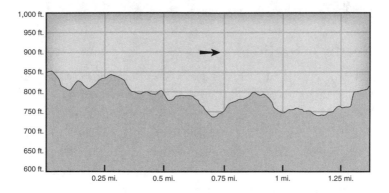

awesome views of Lake Norman. From the trailhead, turn right on the trail, and stay straight. On the left side of the trail you pass a spigot with a dog bowl for the thirsty mutt. This trail is pet-friendly, and dogs are allowed as long as they are on a leash that is no longer than 6 feet.

After 0.2 mile, veer right (southwest) to continue on an asphalt path through the forest. The path curves around the lakeshore, and after 0.3 mile you reach a sunny and sandy beach. Behind the beach is an open grassy area in a grove of pine trees with picnic tables and barbecue grills.

After 400 feet, the trail curves around to the right. An optional spur trail leads to an observation deck with more good views of Lake Norman. After 0.1 mile you pass through the developed section of the park with restrooms, the park office, picnic pavilion, and an A-frame building with skylights that the trail actually passes through. Follow the paved path along the lakeshore and then back into the shade of the forest. This is a very nice section of the trail, with interpretive plaques that identify and describe the surrounding area's black walnut, hickory, redbud, hackberry, red maple, sycamore, and tulip poplar trees.

Follow the trail 0.5 mile until the path curves sharply to the left, but stay straight (southwest). Continue on the paved path for 400 feet until the trail rejoins the playground and the trailhead at the parking lot on the right (northwest).

Nearby Attractions

The park is encircled on three sides by Lake Norman, and a boat ramp provides access to the lake activities. About 0.5 mile to the west is the Peninsula Golf Club—handy if you're in the mood to hit the links. The 43-acre Ramsey Creek Park, about a mile to the south down West Catawba Road, features more nature trails, another boat ramp, and Lake Norman access, as well as a 3-acre dog park. Concessions and lodging are available in the nearby town of Davidson, about 3 miles to the northeast.

Directions

From the Charlotte city center, take I-277 South to I-77 North at Exit 1C toward Statesville. Follow I-77 for 18.6 miles and then take Exit 28 to US 21 South toward Lake Norman, and follow it for 0.2 mile. Turn left onto East Catawba Avenue and follow it for 1.2 miles. Turn right onto Jetton Road and follow it for 0.4 mile, and then turn into Jetton Park on your left. Drive into Jetton Park and pass the entrance gate. Follow the one-way road to the parking lot in front of the playground, on your left.

7 Latta Plantation: Piedmont Prairie Trail & Mountain Island Lake Loop

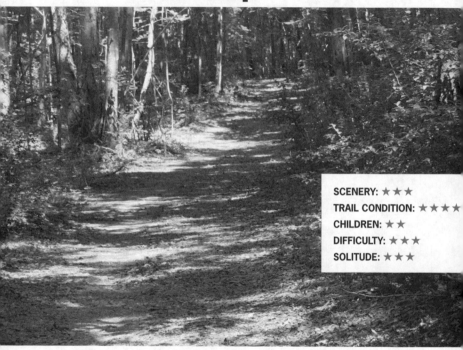

SCENERY: ★ ★ ★
TRAIL CONDITION: ★ ★ ★ ★
CHILDREN: ★ ★
DIFFICULTY: ★ ★ ★
SOLITUDE: ★ ★ ★

A TRAIL IN LATTA PLANTATION EXPLORES A SECTION OF BOTTOMLAND HARDWOOD FOREST

GPS TRAILHEAD COORDINATES: N35° 21.518' W80° 55.026'

DISTANCE & CONFIGURATION: 5.1-mile balloon

HIKING TIME: 3.5 hours

HIGHLIGHTS: Piedmont prairie restoration site, Mountain Island Lake, and bottomland forest

ELEVATION: 660' at the trailhead to 756'

ACCESS: Daily, 7 a.m.–sunset

MAPS: At the Latta Plantation Nature Center and **parkandrec.com**

FACILITIES: Restrooms, nature center, equestrian center, picnic areas, fishing piers, and swimming areas

WHEELCHAIR ACCESS: None

COMMENTS: Of the 16 miles of trails, 13 miles are open to hikers and horses, and 3 miles are designated as hiking-only. Dogs on leashes 6 feet or shorter are welcome.

CONTACTS: (704) 875-1391; **lattaplantation.org**

Overview

The 1,345-acre Latta Plantation Nature Preserve offers an abundance of outdoor activities that include paddling, horseback riding, fishing, birding, and hiking. Along the trails, you will encounter several picnic shelters and fishing piers, so feel free to pack a lunch or bring your pole along for the hike. During the summer, you'd do well to bring along some bug spray. This hike combines several existing trails within the preserve, creating a route that includes most of the highlights of this popular destination. The trail starts in a shady and dense bottomland hardwood forest along the shore of Mountain Island Lake. It skirts past one of the region's few remaining and restored Piedmont prairies (described later) and follows along the shore of Mountain Island Lake, where you will find several small beaches. This trail is best in the spring, before the heat hits Mecklenburg County, or in the fall, when the leaves in Piedmont country are turning color.

Route Details

The Piedmont Prairie Trailhead, noted by a small wooden sign, is on the eastern side of the parking lot directly behind the parking spaces. From here, a roughly 3-foot-wide path leads into the bottomland hardwood forest.

Note: As you'll be hiking on mixed-use pathways, watch out for your equine friends and make sure to give these animals the right-of-way. Provide at least 10 feet of space between you and any horse, and avoid any sudden movements that might spook the animals.

Once on the trail, you will see that oaks and pines dominate the tree population. Shrubs and beautiful ferns thrive in the dense understory. The trail continues through the forest and crosses three

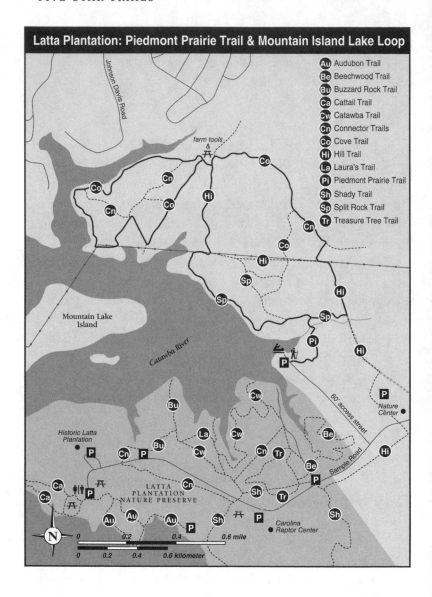

Latta Plantation: Piedmont Prairie Trail & Mountain Island Lake Loop

Au Audubon Trail
Be Beechwood Trail
Bu Buzzard Rock Trail
Ca Cattail Trail
Cw Catawba Trail
Cn Connector Trails
Co Cove Trail
Hi Hill Trail
La Laura's Trail
Pi Piedmont Prairie Trail
Sh Shady Trail
Sp Split Rock Trail
Tr Treasure Tree Trail

small wooden footbridges before running parallel to a small stream that empties into the lake. The very small hills in this section provide some minimal challenge and also raise you to an elevation from which you can view the lake through the forest canopy.

After 0.3 mile you will cross a small stream, but no need to worry about getting your feet wet. Large and stable rocks in the stream provide easy passage. Remain on the Piedmont Prairie Trail for 250 more feet until you reach a junction with the Split Rock Trail. Turn right (east) onto Split Rock Trail. The path here widens into a 4-foot-wide gravel pathway that runs along a rare, restored Piedmont prairie. These Piedmont prairies are believed to have been created by Native Americans who regularly burned their forest areas to keep them open for hunting and agricultural purposes. Today they appear as natural open meadows that harbor a variety of endangered plant species. Here you will find a rare habitat that hosts the endangered Schweinitz's sunflower (*Helianthus schweinitzii*) and Michaux's sumac (*Rhus michauxii*).

At the junction noted above, follow the Split Rock Trail for 0.2 mile and reach a junction for the Hill Trail. Follow the trail for 0.3 mile, turning left (north) onto the gravel road that continues to

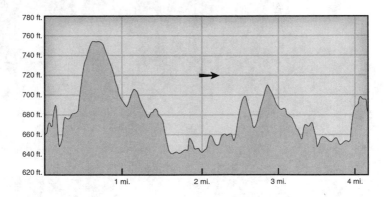

border the Piedmont Prairie, climbing a short hill, and then following the trail as it curves to the left (west). After 0.4 mile you will take a narrow dirt connector trail right (northwest). Follow the connector trail for 300 feet, passing through bottomland hardwood forest, and turn right (north) onto Cove Trail. During this next section you will follow the Cove Trail for 1.2 miles, passing a small picnic table beside a few relic farm tools, winding through bottomland forest, rejoining the shoreline of Mountain Island Lake, and then returning to the picnic table and farm tools. When you reach the picnic table and farm tools, turn right (southeast) onto the Hill Trail again and continue toward the nature center.

Stay on the Hill Trail, going south for 0.4 mile until you reach Split Rock Trail. Turn right (west) here and hike back down to the lakeshore. Along this stretch of trail you will pass four small sandy beaches that are perfect for a swim, a picnic, or just a leisurely break

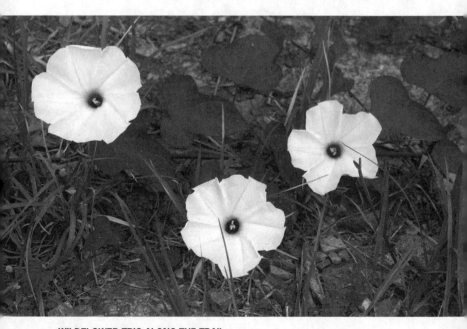

WILDFLOWER TRIO ALONG THE TRAIL

where you can take in the lake view and the surrounding forest. Also along this stretch, you will find a few mature oak and pine trees that escaped the selective harvesting that occurred in this forest. Stay on Split Rock Trail for 0.7 mile, and then turn right (south) back onto Piedmont Prairie Trail. After 0.3 mile you will return to the trailhead and parking lot.

Nearby Attractions

When visiting Latta Plantation Preserve, make sure to check out its historic 19th-century Federal-style plantation home and living museum. The home and grounds are open for interpretive tours. Other attractions include a nature center where you can learn about the native animals of the area and attend interpretive talks at the outdoor amphitheater. The Backyard Habitat Garden, which includes a bird-feeding area, butterfly garden, and a garden pond, is interesting to explore. Also on the preserve is the Carolina Raptor Center, a rehabilitation facility dedicated to the conservation of birds of prey and home to the Southeast's largest eagle aviary. And the Latta Plantation Equestrian Center offers guided horseback rides, horse shows, and lessons in horse care and riding.

Directions

From the Charlotte city center, travel north on I-77 and take Exit 18/W. T. Harris Boulevard. Turn left and drive 1.7 miles to Mt. Holly–Huntersville Road. Turn left and drive 1.2 miles. Turn right on Beatties Ford Road. Drive 1.5 miles north and turn left onto Sample Road. Continue 1 mile and arrive at the preserve entrance on your left, which is marked by a stone wall and a small brown sign. Follow Sample Road past the nature center and turn right on the next paved road toward the canoe launch and trailhead. The road turns from pavement to gravel and continues down to the lakeshore. Park your vehicle on the left side of the lot. The trailhead is on the right side of the parking lot.

8

South Mountains State Park: High Shoals Falls Loop

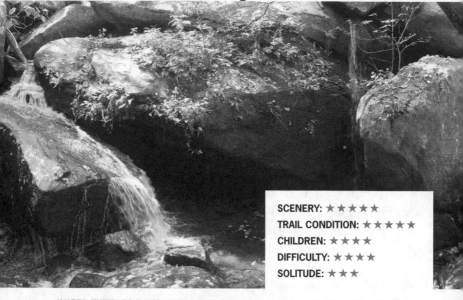

SCENERY: ★ ★ ★ ★ ★
TRAIL CONDITION: ★ ★ ★ ★ ★
CHILDREN: ★ ★ ★ ★
DIFFICULTY: ★ ★ ★ ★
SOLITUDE: ★ ★

WATER TUMBLES DOWN THE JACOB FORK RIVER ALONG THE HIGH SHOALS FALLS LOOP.

GPS TRAILHEAD COORDINATES: N35° 36.135' W81° 37.766'

DISTANCE & CONFIGURATION: 2.4-mile balloon

HIKING TIME: 2 hours

HIGHLIGHTS: High Shoals Falls, mature forest, mountain views, Shinny Creek, and Jacob Fork River

ELEVATION: 1,374' at the trailhead to 1,943'

ACCESS: November–February: Daily, 8 a.m.–6 p.m.; March–April and September–October: Daily, 8 a.m.–8 p.m.; May–August: Daily, 8 a.m.–9 p.m.; permits needed for camping; Cicero Campground and backcountry sites $13 per night

MAPS: At the visitor center, the trailhead kiosk, and ncparks.gov, but those map scales are too small for detailed depictions; the nature center sells a much better and highly recommended U.S. Geological Survey topo map.

FACILITIES: Restrooms, water fountains, picnic pavilions, horse facilities, and amphi-theater; the visitor center provides permits for the campgrounds and for backcountry camping.

WHEELCHAIR ACCESS: Only at the visitor center and at the beginning of the trail, which is paved, and to the picnic area about 20 yards from the trailhead

COMMENTS: To avoid crowds at this very popular destination, come during the week and avoid holidays. If you're going to hike only one trail in this entire book, this is it. It's moderately challenging, so if you don't like climbing, you might want to rethink hiking it. However, I highly encourage you to try it.

CONTACTS: (828) 433-4772; **ncparks.gov**

Overview

The trail really has everything you can hope for in a hike around Charlotte. You start off on level ground and follow alongside a very beautiful and rocky creek. It's very picturesque and surrounded by a wonderfully mature and healthy, leafy forest. From here the trail begins to climb gradually and crosses several very well-constructed bridges. Along the way there are ample boulder-filled creek passages that scream "photo op," and small clearings and a rocky shoreline that have "picnic" and "cloud watching" written all over them. The path really starts to climb once you reach a series of wooden staircases. The good part, besides the physical challenge of the endeavor, is that the staircases wind over a cascading creek and lead to the trail's highlight: an 80-foot waterfall. From here the trail descends somewhat steeply back down to the gently rolling river and welcomed level ground. It's really a wonderful and stimulating trail that shouldn't be missed, but if you have a hard time getting up the steps in a two-story house, then this isn't the trail for you.

Route Details

At the west end of the paved lot, a large kiosk and a short wooden walkway mark the trailhead to the High Shoals Falls Loop. There's a lot of uphill and downhill, so you may want to bring a hiking stick or some trekking poles. Follow the 4-foot-wide paved path into the forest. After 300 feet, a spur trail to the left (south) leads to a picnic area, but stay straight (west) and pass that area.

Immediately after the picnic area and before the path becomes a 10-foot-wide gravel path, it skirts a small rustic cabin that houses

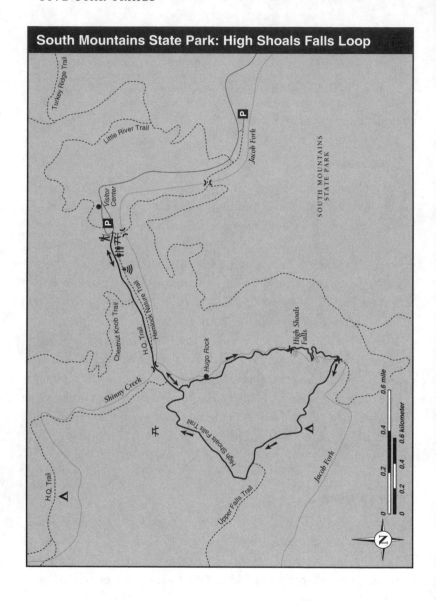

South Mountains State Park: High Shoals Falls Loop

restrooms. After 0.1 mile, the trail passes wooden steps on the left (south) that lead to the amphitheater at the bottom of the hill. Stay straight (west) and continue on the blue circle–blazed High Shoals Falls Loop. After 300 feet, you reach the Chestnut Knob Trail. Stay straight (west) on the High Shoals Falls Loop and continue toward the falls that are 0.8 mile from this junction. Meanwhile, in 0.1 mile, you will reach the junction with the Hemlock Nature Trail on the left (south). But stay straight (west) on the High Shoals Falls Loop.

Shortly after the junction with the Hemlock Nature Trail, you cross a small wooden bridge that spans beautiful Shinny Creek. On the other side of the masterfully constructed bridge is the Shinny Creek picnic area, with tables set in a large, shaded, and picturesque clearing. Cut across the clearing and continue on the High Shoals Falls Loop. About 20 yards after the picnic area, you reach the junction with the Shinny Creek Campsite Trail on the right (northwest). Stay straight (southwest) on the High Shoals Falls Loop that ascends a series of wooden steps and then follows alongside Shinny Creek. After 0.1 mile you reach a curious patch of broken slab rocks that cover the trail. This is known as Hugo Rock. The rocks found their way down the mountain during a rockslide caused by erosion during the violently powerful

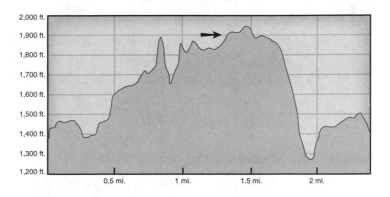

Hurricane Hugo in 1989. Here is an impressive display of the power of the storm and of the impacts erosion can have on the landscape.

After Hugo Rock, the trail passes over a small wooden footbridge and crosses through large boulders and rock formations before it reaches the long series of wooden staircases that lead to the waterfalls. The stairs climb over a series of cascading falls tumbling over large boulders. From here you gain 190 feet of elevation over the next 490 feet of trail, reaching an observation deck at the foot of an impressive 80-foot waterfall, the highlight of the trail.

After enjoying the wonderful sight of the falls, turn around and continue on the High Shoals Falls Loop, turning right (southeast) to continue up the staircase. From here the trail is very easy to follow. The staircase continues up to a ridge where you have fantastic views of the surrounding mountains before gradually descending, crossing the Jacob Fork River via a wooden railed bridge and continuing to the junction with the Upper Falls Trail. Turn right (northeast) onto the High Shoals Falls Loop toward the rustic fence. From here the trail climbs over a series of small hills for the next 0.5 mile and then really starts a steep descent back to rejoin Shinny Creek. In just 0.3 mile the trail descends a steep 580 feet and reaches Shinny Creek and the beginning of the loop section of the hike, which you will reach at the bottom of the descent. To the right (south) the trail leads back to Hugo Rock and the waterfalls route that you have already traversed. Here, you will turn left (northeast) and continue on the conjoined High Shoals Falls Loop and Hemlock Nature Trail. Simply stay straight (northeast) on the High Shoals Falls Loop for 0.4 mile, climbing over one last hill and then ascending to the trailhead, parking lot, and the end of the hike.

Nearby Attractions

South Mountains State Park, in Connelly Springs, North Carolina, is 67 miles northwest of Downtown Charlotte and is hands-down the best park within an hour's drive from the city center. There really aren't many reasons to go anywhere else, as the park has more than

40 miles of really impressive and well-maintained hiking trails, most of them dotted with backcountry campsites along the routes if you want to get out in the park for an extended backpacking trip. Plan to spend some time at the visitor center. It offers awesome displays of the area's wildlife and provides microscopes for close-ups at some of the park's insects and microscopic organisms. Hickory, North Carolina, known as the furniture capital, is a great place for provisions and dining just 11 miles or 15 minutes to the northeast of the park.

Directions

South Mountains State Park is in Burke County, 20.5 miles south of Morganton. From I-40, turn south on NC 18 at Exit 105, travel 11.1 miles, and make a right turn onto NC 1913 (Sugarloaf Road). Take NC 1913 4.3 miles to Old NC 18 and turn left. Travel 2.7 miles and make a right turn onto NC 1901 (Ward Gap Road). The park is 1.4 miles off NC 1901 on NC 1904 (South Mountain Park Avenue). Travel 1 mile from the beginning of South Mountain Park Avenue to the South Mountains State Park gate. Drive west down the park's main paved road, South Mountain Park Avenue. You'll pass the visitor center and roadside campground, then continue to the large parking lot at the very end of the avenue.

9

South Mountains State Park: River Trail

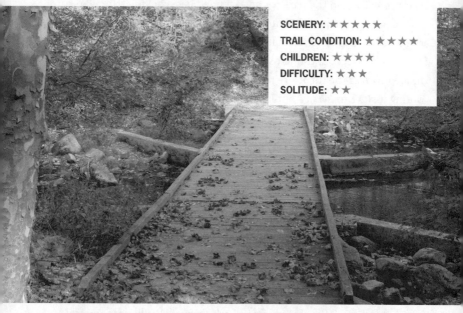

SCENERY: ★ ★ ★ ★ ★
TRAIL CONDITION: ★ ★ ★ ★ ★
CHILDREN: ★ ★ ★ ★
DIFFICULTY: ★ ★ ★
SOLITUDE: ★ ★

A LEAF-LITTERED BRIDGE SPANS THE JACOB FORK RIVER.

GPS TRAILHEAD COORDINATES: N35° 36.126' W81° 37.763'

DISTANCE & CONFIGURATION: 1.7-mile loop

HIKING TIME: 1.5 hours

HIGHLIGHTS: Jacob Fork River

ELEVATION: 1,454' at the trailhead to 1,696'

ACCESS: November–February: Daily, 8 a.m.–6 p.m.; March–April and September–October: Daily, 8 a.m.–8 p.m.; May–August: Daily, 8 a.m.–9 p.m.; permits needed for camping; Cicero Campground and backcountry sites $13 per night

MAPS: At the visitor center, the trailhead kiosk, and ncparks.gov, but those map scales are too small for detailed depictions; the nature center sells a much better and highly recommended U.S. Geological Survey topo map.

FACILITIES: Restrooms, water fountains, picnic pavilions, horse facilities, and amphitheater; the visitor center provides permits for the campgrounds and for backcountry camping.

WHEELCHAIR ACCESS: Only at the visitor center and at the beginning of the trail, which is paved, and to the picnic area about 20 yards from the trailhead.

COMMENTS: To avoid crowds at this very popular destination, come during the week, and avoid holidays. This trail is highly recommended and is situated in one of the nicest parks within an hour's drive of Charlotte.

CONTACTS: (828) 433-4772; **ncparks.gov**

Overview

This route combines three trails—the River Trail, Raven Rock Trail, and Little River Trail—to create a loop in South Mountains State Park. The route starts on the River Trail and follows along the picturesque bank of the Jacob Fork River. Plenty of picnic areas and inspiringly restful spots are along the way. From here the trail ascends some moderate elevation on the Raven Rock Trail, offering views of the surrounding mountains, and descends on the Little River Trail to the parking lot where you started. The hike offers a bit of challenge interspersed with beautiful forest and wonderful riverside walking.

Route Details

A large kiosk and a wooden bridge at the southwest corner of the parking lot mark the trailhead to the River Trail, which is blazed with red triangles. Cross over the footbridge that spans the Jacob Fork River and continue down the River Trail alongside the water. On this pleasantly level section you will come to several small, flat, grassy clearings along the riverbank. You may want to pause and take in the sound and sights of the water rolling through the leafy forest, around boulders, and over rocks.

Continue on the gradually descending River Trail for 0.4 mile to the junction with the Upper Falls Trail. Turn left (east), remaining on the River Trail and crossing another wooden footbridge over the Jacob Fork River.

The River Trail follows alongside Jacob Fork for another 400 feet before arriving at the trail junction with the Family Campground Trail. Turn left (northeast) following the 10-foot-wide, gravel Raven Rock Trail uphill. The Raven Rock Trail is marked with white circular blazes. After about 30 yards, the trail arrives at the paved South

South Mountains State Park: River Trail

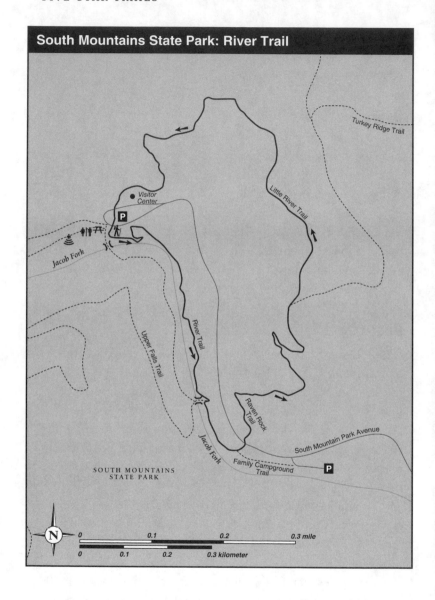

Turkey Ridge Trail

Little River Trail

Visitor Center

Jacob Fork

Upper Falls Trail

River Trail

Raven Rock Trail

South Mountain Park Avenue

Jacob Fork

Family Campground Trail

SOUTH MOUNTAINS STATE PARK

N

| 0 | 0.1 | 0.2 | 0.3 mile |

| 0 | 0.1 | 0.2 | 0.3 kilometer |

Mountain Park Avenue. Cross the road and continue climbing steeply uphill for 0.4 mile on a series of switchbacks that ascend 385 feet and offer fantastic views of the surrounding mountains. After the climb, you reach the junction with the Little River Trail. Turn left (north) onto the Little River Trail, blazed with blue triangles, and continue climbing uphill for 0.1 more mile before beginning a very gradual descent. From this junction the trail is very easy to follow. The route descends 413 feet over the next 0.7 mile and ends at the trailhead, in the northwest corner of the parking lot where you started.

Nearby Attractions

South Mountains State Park, in Connelly Springs, North Carolina, is 67 miles northwest of Downtown Charlotte and is hands-down the best park within an hour's drive from the city center. The history of South Mountains State Park is very interesting. Before the 18,000 acres of rugged mountains were designated as a state park, they were used as major travel routes and farming lands by the early European settlers. Earlier than that, they served as a buffer zone between the warring Cherokee and Catawba Native Americans. Gold

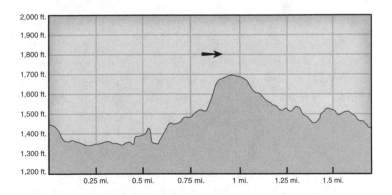

was discovered in 1828 when a frontiersman found glittering flakes in the mud he was using to seal his log cabin. A gold rush ensued, flooding the area with settlers and prospectors, until the gold was mostly mined and the operations ceased around 1900.

Like many of the eastern U.S. national and state parks, South Mountains State Park was originally a Civilian Conservation Corps work camp during the Great Depression. In fact, the CCC built most of the park's bridges, towers, and buildings. The park's highest peak is Buzzards Roost, which rises to 3,000 feet in elevation. Most of the trails in the park offer spectacular views of the surrounding mountains. I highly recommend exploring more of the trails in this wonderful park.

There really aren't many reasons to go anywhere else, as the park has more than 40 miles of very impressive and well-maintained hiking trails, most of them dotted with backcountry campsites along the routes if you want to get out in the park for an extended backpacking trip. Hickory, North Carolina, known as the furniture capital, is a great place for provisions and dining just 11 miles or 15 minutes to the northeast of the park.

Directions

South Mountains State Park is in Burke County, 20.5 miles south of Morganton. From I-40, turn south on NC 18 at Exit 105. Travel 11.1 miles, and make a right turn onto NC 1913 (Sugarloaf Road). Take NC 1913 4.3 miles to Old NC 18 and turn left. Travel 2.7 miles and make a right turn onto NC 1901 (Ward Gap Road). The park is 1.4 miles off NC 1901 on NC 1904 (South Mountain Park Avenue). Travel 1 mile from the beginning of South Mountain Park Avenue to the South Mountains State Park gate. Drive west down the park's main paved road, South Mountain Park Avenue. You'll pass the visitor center and roadside campground, then continue to the large parking lot at the very end of the avenue.

10

Torrence Creek Greenway East

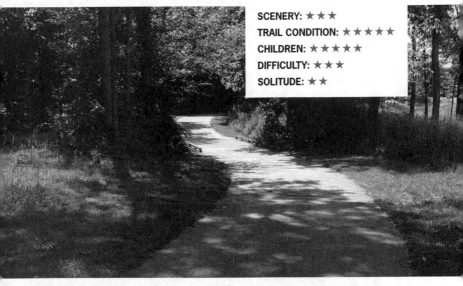

SCENERY: ★ ★ ★
TRAIL CONDITION: ★ ★ ★ ★ ★
CHILDREN: ★ ★ ★ ★ ★
DIFFICULTY: ★ ★ ★
SOLITUDE: ★ ★

THE WELL-MAINTAINED PATHS OF TORRENCE CREEK GREENWAY EAST MAKE THIS TRAIL AN EXCELLENT CHOICE FOR RUNNERS AND HIKERS.

GPS TRAILHEAD COORDINATES: Bradford Hill Lane Trailhead: N35° 24.212' W80° 52.983'

DISTANCE & CONFIGURATION: 1.7-mile out-and-back

HIKING TIME: 2 hours

HIGHLIGHTS: Torrence Creek and rock formations

ELEVATION: 675' at the trailhead to 712'

ACCESS: Daily, sunrise–sunset

MAPS: At Charlotte Visitor Info Center and **parkandrec.com**

FACILITIES: None

WHEELCHAIR ACCESS: Yes, along paved portions of trails

COMMENTS: Trail is shared with bikers, runners, and inline skaters. Dogs are allowed on leashes 6 feet or shorter.

CONTACTS: (704) 432-1369; **parkandrec.com**

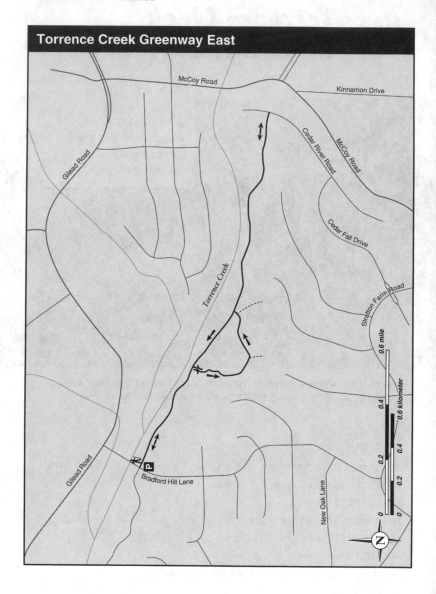

Torrence Creek Greenway East

Overview

In Huntersville, North Carolina, about 20 minutes from Charlotte's city center, the Torrence Creek Greenway is ideal for a leisurely jog, a bike ride, or an afternoon walk with children or pets. The greenway, accessible from the on-street parking on Bradford Hill Lane, runs alongside its namesake creek through wetlands and forested terrain, and several very interesting, large rock formations are found along the path. The trail surface combines a paved path with a boardwalk and wooden footbridges and also includes a few short sections of gravel at the east end of the greenway.

Route Details

The Torrence Creek Greenway is clearly marked with gray-and-blue CHARMECK PARKS AND RECREATION signs where the greenway crosses Bradford Hill Lane. Enter onto the greenway on the east side of the road. This greenway is largely used as a pedestrian footpath connecting different neighborhoods in the area, but it's popular with runners and bikers, so be aware that you'll be sharing the paved trail. Several grassy clearings make for a nice place to throw down a blanket and relax along the creek and the trail. Please note that there are no water fountains or other suitable drinking sources along this trail, so make sure to bring water along with you on this hike.

The paved path runs alongside Torrence Creek, through a young forest, then crosses a small wooden footbridge. During the summer and spring, wildflowers bloom along the trail's edge, where sunlight breaks through the forest canopy in the swath clearing that the trail has created. On this section of the greenway, observe the restoration work done to battle erosion on the bank of the creek. The textured-concrete molded stones have a gray-and-pink tone that blends well into the natural environment; soon plants will begin to grow again along the bank, and the stones that secure the bank soil will blend in well and hardly be noticed by those using this greenway.

After 0.2 mile you reach a junction in the trail. Turn right (south) onto the more narrow paved spur trail, where you cross another small wooden footbridge. During this section you will want to stay on the paved trails. The dirt and gravel trails that you encounter lead to homes or back onto neighborhood streets.

Continue for 0.1 mile until the trail splits in two directions. Stay to the left (east). The trail to the right leads back into the neighborhood. Stay on the paved path and cross the wooden bridge ahead. The trail passes by several homes before reaching another junction where you keep left (east). Here you pass the first group of large rock formations that seem oddly out of place in the forest, causing you to wonder how in the world they got here. However, they have probably always been here, and erosion has simply uncovered or created them. Continue along the paved trail and climb the small hill passing through another cluster of exceptionally large boulders.

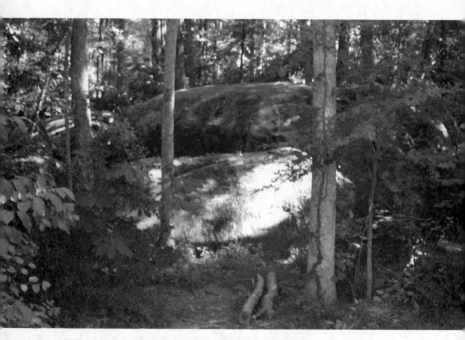

ONE OF THE TRAIL'S SIGNATURE BOULDER FORMATIONS

Some of these rock formations are as big as a school bus. They are truly amazing, and kids will really get a kick out of them. Some of the rock formations have flat surfaces that make a great place to sit. The neighborhood is fairly quiet and the sound of Torrence Creek is enough to create a very calming environment. After 0.4 mile the trail ends at the top of the hill once you reach Cedar River Road. From here, turn around and follow the greenway alongside Torrence Creek. Continue back the way you came for 0.4 mile until you arrive back at the intersection where you first turned right. Stay straight (west) along the paved path and continue straight along the greenway back to the trailhead on Bradford Hill Lane.

Nearby Attractions

Lake Norman is accessible along NC 73 by heading about 3 miles northwest toward Hicks Crossroads. Jetton Park (see pages 50 and 55), on Lake Norman, features additional trails and facilities. It's 6 miles north along Catawba Avenue just off I-77. Amenities and concessions are available in Huntersville, just 2 miles to the east on Gilead Road. The 1,300-acre Latta Plantation (see page 60), a historic cotton plantation and living-history museum in Huntersville, offers 16 miles of trails, a raptor center, and an equestrian facility. I highly recommend it.

Directions

From the Charlotte city center, take I-277 South and then merge onto I-77 North at Exit 1C toward Statesville for 13.2 miles. Take the Gilead Road exit, Exit 23, toward Huntersville. Turn right onto Gilead Road and follow it for 0.3 mile. Here, Gilead Road bears left. Turn left and continue to follow Gilead Road for 1.6 miles. Turn left onto Bradford Hill Lane and follow it for 0.6 mile. Park alongside Bradford Hill Lane on the left side of the road.

University Research Park Trail

SCENERY: ★ ★ ★
TRAIL CONDITION: ★ ★ ★ ★ ★
CHILDREN: ★ ★ ★
DIFFICULTY: ★ ★
SOLITUDE: ★ ★ ★

MALLARD CREEK RUNS BESIDE THE UNIVERSITY RESEARCH PARK TRAIL.

GPS TRAILHEAD COORDINATES: N35° 19.584' W80° 46.371'

DISTANCE & CONFIGURATION: 2.7-mile out-and-back

HIKING TIME: 2 hours

HIGHLIGHTS: Hardwood forest and Mallard Creek

ELEVATION: 632' at the trailhead to 599' at lowest point

ACCESS: 24/7 but not recommended after dark due to the isolation of the trail

MAPS: At Charlotte Visitor Info Center and **parkandrec.com**

FACILITIES: None

WHEELCHAIR ACCESS: None

COMMENTS: Leashed dogs allowed on leashes 6 feet or shorter. Hikers share the trail with bikers, runners, inline skaters, and skateboarders.

CONTACTS: (704) 432-1570; **parkandrec.com**

Overview

This trail follows a 1.2-mile section of the much larger 7.1-mile-long Clark's Creek and Mallard Creek Greenway through the Charlotte University Research Park. The research park, operated by the University of North Carolina at Charlotte, and used for research in horticulture and environmental-science projects. Don't be surprised if you encounter a few students or professors collecting data along the trail. This route begins at the Countryside Montessori School and runs through a beautiful mature pine-and-hardwood forest before ending at Research Drive. The trail is great for running and biking, and on each side of the trail is a soft, grassy swath that is exceptionally easy on the knees.

Route Details

I recommend that you hike this trail outside of school hours during the week or on weekends, but if you're here during school hours, it's a good idea to let someone know that you are here to hike the trail by visiting the front office. It can be hot out here on this trail during the summer, as quite a bit of the trail is exposed to the sun. Make sure to bring plenty of water to drink if you're here during a hotter part of the year.

To get to the trail, walk along the outside of the fence of the school's playground and sports field. Directly behind the playground is a paved path. Turn left (east) onto the paved path toward the research park section of the Clark's Creek and Mallard Creek Greenway.

The 6-foot-wide trail is in very good condition. Follow it for about 0.1 mile, under power lines and through a cleared swath that stretches north to south. Here the pavement ends and the trail becomes gravel, entering into the shade of a more mature hardwood forest. Follow the trail around the bend to the left. It is a wide and easy trail to follow; just stay on the gravel. The trail, which connects quite a few neighborhoods, is good for bikes and ideal for running or speed walking.

University Research Park Trail

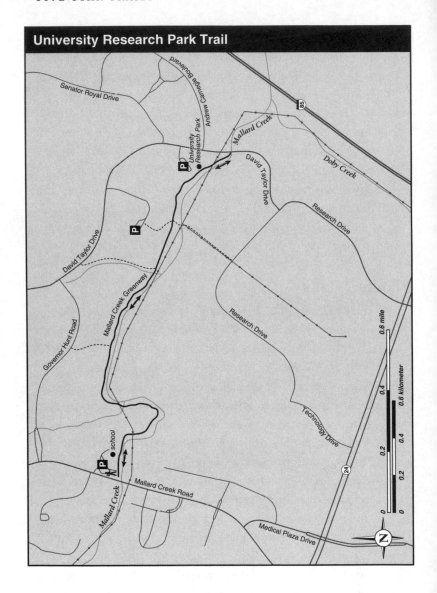

Continue on the trail for another 0.2 mile, where it begins to follow alongside the wide and rocky Mallard Creek. The creek is shallow in the summer except after the heavy afternoon thunderstorms that occur frequently during this time of year. After 0.3 mile from where the trail meets with the creek, the trail splits to the left. Continue straight (east). The left spur leads to Governor Hunt Road. This trail is not recommended after dark due to the isolated nature of the trail, but during daylight hours police officers on motorcycles patrol it and provide an exceptional element of safety along the route. At this point in the trail, the forest canopy really opens up as the trail begins to follow a cleared swath of land for power lines.

Continue along the trail for 0.3 mile until you come to the next junction, where the trail splits off to the left again. This time the spur trail leads to David Taylor Drive and back into the neighborhood there. Stay straight (east) along the main trail for 0.1 mile until you come to a crossroads or four-way split in the trail. Stay straight again on the main trail, going toward the chain-link fence and passing the metal bridge on your left that leads to Research Drive. Soon the trail thankfully enters back into the shade of the forest. Pass the large brick building on your left before arriving at Research Drive and the end of the research park section of Clark's Creek and Mallard Creek Greenway. Research Drive can come up on you quickly, so be prepared if you are hiking with a pet. Here you can turn around and hike back the way you came in and return to the parking lot at Countryside Montessori School.

Nearby Attractions

The research-park walk is very close to the University of North Carolina at Charlotte. At the university, just 4 miles to the southeast, you can find more hiking trails at the very impressive botanical gardens (see page 110). Also just 6 miles to the southeast is the 737-acre Reedy Creek Nature Preserve (see page 105), with hiking and walking trails, a nature center with a museum and gardens, and two ponds that are open for fishing.

Directions

From the Charlotte city center, take I-277 South/US 74 West and merge onto I-77 North/US 21 North via Exit 1C toward Statesville and follow it for 3.4 miles. Merge onto I-85 North via Exit 13A toward Greensboro and follow it for 6.5 miles. Merge onto NC 24 West/W. T. Harris Boulevard via Exit 45B and follow it for 1.5 miles. Turn right onto Mallard Creek Road and follow it for 0.7 mile. Countryside Montessori School will be on your right, at 9026 Mallard Creek Road. Park your vehicle at the school, in the back of the parking lot near the baseball field.

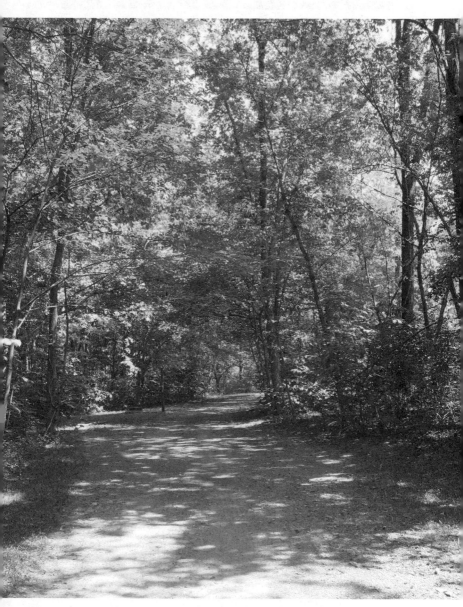

A SUN-DAPPLED STRETCH OF THE UNIVERSITY RESEARCH PARK TRAIL

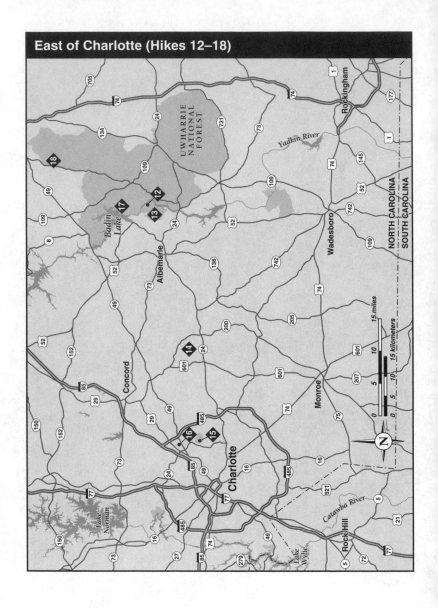

East of Charlotte (Hikes 12–18)

East of Charlotte

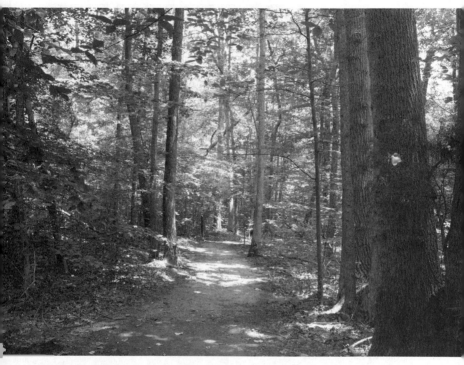

THE TRAILS OF REEDY CREEK NATURE PRESERVE EXPLORE HARDWOOD
FORESTS SUCH AS THE ONE SHOWN HERE.

Morrow Mountain State Park: Fall Mountain Trail

SCENERY: ★ ★ ★ ★ ★
TRAIL CONDITION: ★ ★ ★
CHILDREN: ★ ★
DIFFICULTY: ★ ★ ★ ★
SOLITUDE: ★ ★ ★

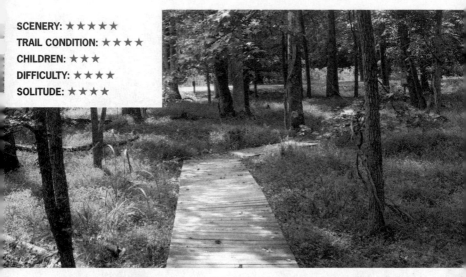

WOODEN BOARDWALKS AT THE BEGINNING OF THE TRAIL TRAVERSE BEAUTIFUL LOW-LYING FOREST LAND ON THE FLOODPLAIN OF THE YADKIN RIVER.

GPS TRAILHEAD COORDINATES: N35° 22.887' W80° 3.764'

DISTANCE & CONFIGURATION: 4.0-mile loop

HIKING TIME: 3.5 hours

HIGHLIGHTS: Fall Mountain, Yadkin River, and challenging hills

ELEVATION: 297' at the trailhead to 723'

ACCESS: November–February: Daily, 8 a.m.–6 p.m.; March–May and September–October: Daily, 8 a.m.–8 p.m.; June–August: Daily, 8 a.m.–9 p.m.; cabin rental $88 per night; campsites with electricity $20 per night

MAPS: At the park's visitor center, trailhead kiosks, and **ncparks.gov**

FACILITIES: Restrooms, water spigots, boat launch, rental cabins, campground for tent and RV use, amphitheater, and picnic pavilions

WHEELCHAIR ACCESS: Some of the park trails and areas are wheelchair-accessible, but this trail is not.

COMMENTS: This trail makes quite a climb up Fall Mountain, so allow for more hiking time than you would for many of the other easier trails in this book.

CONTACTS: (704) 982-4402; **ncparks.gov**

Overview

The trail starts in the northeast section of the park, departing from the parking lot for the boat launch on the Yadkin River. This exceptionally beautiful and equally challenging hike is not to be missed. If you choose to do only a handful of trails in this book, I would highly recommend hiking this trail. After leaving the parking lot, the trail begins to ascend quickly and steeply. The trail climbs to the top of Fall Mountain, where, were it not for the very beautiful forest surrounding the trail, you would possibly be disappointed that the views were not better. You get to steal a few far-reaching views through the trees, and more in the wintertime, before the trail descends steeply back down to the wide Yadkin River. The trail follows along the river shore for more than 0.5 mile. This section is very beautiful and enjoyable, not to mention comfortably level. Even if you don't want to climb Fall Mountain, do this trail in reverse and just hike the level portion along the river. You'll be glad you did. The challenging hills and climb to Fall Mountain make this trail an exceptional choice for fitness training, preparing for longer backpacking trips, and trying out new hiking gear before you take it on long expeditions.

Route Details

A large brown sign in the southwest corner of the parking lot marks the Fall Mountain Trailhead. Follow the 2-foot-wide dirt path blazed with orange triangles over a series of wooden boardwalks before veering to the right (northwest). The trail crosses a gravel road and starts the long climb uphill. The trail is easy to follow and well marked but at times is not very well maintained. In several areas, downed trees lie across the trail and you have to climb over them or follow paths around the obstacles. The trail climbs a steep hill, ascending 136 feet in less than 0.25 mile until the path reaches a second gravel road. The trail descends to a creek before continuing through a very hilly section with steep climbs up to the top of Fall Mountain, where you'll climb 337 feet in about 0.75 mile. I hope you have your hiking boots

Morrow Mountain State Park: Fall Mountain Trail

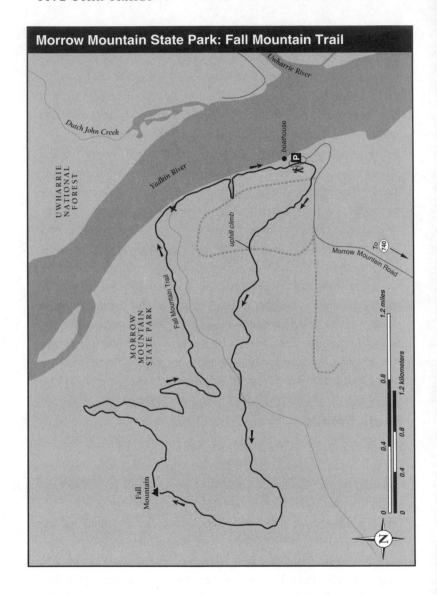

on for this one! The section of trail ascending to Fall Mountain is well maintained. The path climbs until it veers right (west) and then levels out on top of Fall Mountain's ridge. There are no real spectacular views up here, but occasionally you see some of the other surrounding ridges through the trees. The level ground offers a nice break from the hard climb behind you. After you walk through mature forest on the ridge for 0.3 mile, the trail veers right (east) and begins a gradual descent to the Yadkin River. Along this section, lots of large boulders and rocks make the setting feel especially mountainous. The trail follows a short series of switchbacks and is pretty easy coasting downhill for the next 0.5 mile until the trail reaches the Yadkin, where the path follows along the river's edge. This section of the trail is fairly level, with trees arching over the path and lining the river, providing a leafy and shaded walk with excellent views across the river. It's really beautiful. After 0.6 mile, the trail reaches a small bit of land that juts out into the river. Turn right (southwest) and follow the trail across a wooden bridge over a small moving creek. The trail continues along the river's edge for another 0.2 mile until it reaches a small creek that feeds into the river. The trail takes a short detour around the creek,

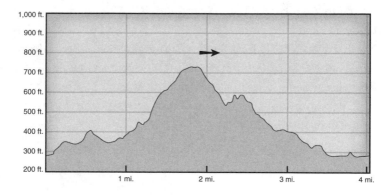

turning right (west). Cross the creek via a gravel road, and then follow the trail along the other side of the creek and back to the river shore. Follow the trail for another 0.2 mile until it reaches the boathouse, the north side of the parking lot, and the northern trailhead.

Nearby Attractions

Morrow Mountain State Park has more than 15 miles of hiking trails to explore, many of them very well maintained and traversing exceptionally beautiful forests filled with plenty of winding streams. Some of the mountain trails offer views of the surrounding mountains and farmlands; the best view is on Morrow Mountain, which is accessible by a road and has a paved parking lot at its peak. The Uwharrie National Forest (see pages 115 and 121) is 20 minutes to the east around Troy, North Carolina, with many more hiking and recreation opportunities. You can also explore the very cool (literally) underground trails of the Reed Gold Mine (see page 100), the site of historic ore veins, 40 minutes to the west in Midland, North Carolina.

Directions

From the Charlotte city center, merge onto US 74 East toward NC 27 and follow it for 3.8 miles. Merge onto NC 27 East via Exit 246 on the left and follow it for 38.2 miles. NC 27 East becomes NC 740 North. Follow NC 740 for 1.9 miles. Turn right onto Morrow Mountain Road/NC 1798. Continue to follow Morrow Mountain Road for 2.8 miles, where you reach the entrance to Morrow Mountain State Park. Follow the signs to the boat-launch parking lot, in the northeast section of the park.

Morrow Mountain State Park: Sugarloaf Mountain Trail

SCENERY: ★ ★ ★ ★
TRAIL CONDITION: ★ ★ ★ ★ ★
CHILDREN: ★ ★ ★
DIFFICULTY: ★ ★ ★ ★
SOLITUDE: ★ ★ ★ ★

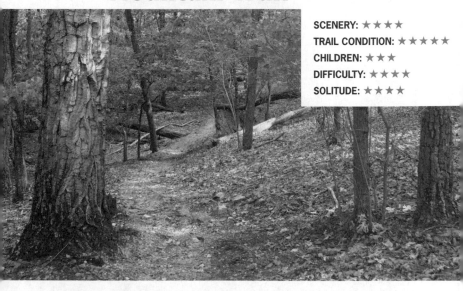

LOOKING FOR A CHALLENGE? HIKE UP SUGARLOAF MOUNTAIN IN MORROW MOUNTAIN STATE PARK.

GPS TRAILHEAD COORDINATES: N35° 21.925' W80° 5.517'

DISTANCE & CONFIGURATION: 2.8-mile loop

HIKING TIME: 2.5 hours

HIGHLIGHTS: Sugarloaf Mountain and challenging hills

ELEVATION: 550' at the trailhead to 869'

ACCESS: November–February: Daily, 8 a.m.–6 p.m.; March–May and September–October: Daily, 8 a.m.–8 p.m.; June–August: Daily, 8 a.m.–9 p.m.; cabin rental $88 per night; campsites with electricity $20 per night

MAPS: At the park's visitor center, trailhead kiosks, and **ncparks.gov**

FACILITIES: Restrooms, water spigots, boat launch, rental cabins, campground for tent and RV use, amphitheater, and picnic pavilions

WHEELCHAIR ACCESS: Some of the park trails and areas are wheelchair-accessible, but this trail is not.

COMMENTS: This trail makes quite a climb up Sugarloaf Mountain, so allow for more hiking time than you would for many of the other easier trails in this book. Also bring a little more water than usual, especially if it's a hot day.

CONTACTS: (704) 982-4402; **ncparks.gov**

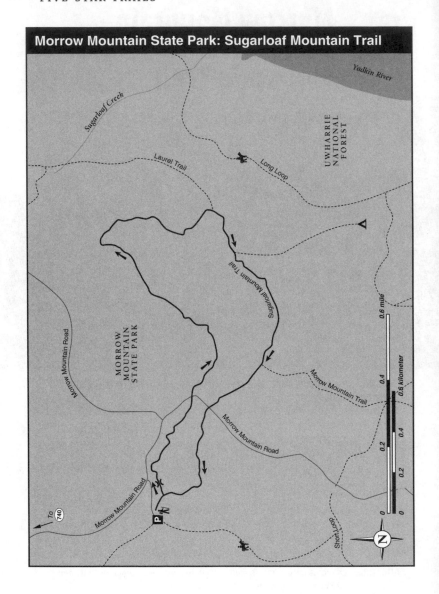

Morrow Mountain State Park: Sugarloaf Mountain Trail

Overview

The Sugarloaf Mountain Trail starts from the horse-trailer parking lot in the southwest section of Morrow Mountain State Park. The trailhead isn't very well marked, so pick up a map at the park's office on your way to the trail, and be sure you know where the trailhead is on the map. The main feature of this trail is the challenging climb up Sugarloaf Mountain. It's some good exercise, and you get to sneak some views through the trees when you get to the top of the mountain. The trail winds through an exceptionally pleasant and beautiful forest. It's a fun loop hike and a good workout that gives you a great overview of what Morrow Mountain State Park has to offer.

Route Details

The trailhead is in the southeastern corner of the horse-trailer parking lot, and the trail is marked with orange diamond-shaped blazes. Follow the 2-foot-wide dirt path for 300 feet until it splits. Stay to the left and follow the trail on the northern part of the loop. The trail follows alongside the road and is fairly level for 0.1 mile; it then starts

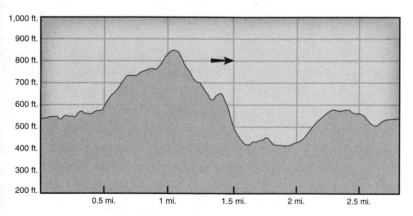

abruptly climbing. The next 0.2 mile climbs 65 feet before descending down to a footbridge crossing a small creek. Continue for 0.2 mile, crossing over a series of small hills, until you reach a paved road. On this section of the trail it is easy to lose the path in the sections with a lot of exposed rock. Keep your eyes open for the orange blazes, and you'll make it through just fine. Once you reach the paved road, continue on the orange-blazed trail on the other side.

This is where the trail really starts to climb. In the next 0.6 mile you will climb 368 feet to the top of Sugarloaf Mountain. It's great fitness or backpacking training. At the top you don't get any spectacular views, but you can see a few of the ridges and surrounding farmland through the trees. Enjoy it because once you reach the top, it's not long before a very steep descent begins. On the climb down, the trail is lined with sometimes arching rhododendrons. This section of the path has a high mountain Appalachian feel. During the descent, you get a few small views of the surrounding ridges and traverse over some sections of loose rocks, otherwise known as scree, so watch your footing on these sections. The trail is steep and can get slick and muddy after rainfall. Watch your step and avoid slipping on the steeper sections as you descend back down the mountain. After 0.5 mile, turn right (southwest), where the Laurel Trail converges with the Sugarloaf Mountain Trail. In 0.3 mile the trail will split again. To the left (south) the trail leads down to a backcountry camping site. Stay to the right (west) and continue along the Sugarloaf Mountain Trail. In 0.2 mile more, the trail intersects with the Morrow Mountain Trail. Stay straight (east) on the Sugarloaf Mountain Trail. From here the trail traverses over a few small hills that are easy compared to the climb you just completed behind you. It's only 0.2 mile to a paved road crossing, where you cross the road and follow the trail on the other side. After 0.4 mile you reach the parking lot and the end of the trail.

Nearby Attractions

Morrow Mountain State Park has more than 15 miles of hiking trails to explore, many of them very well maintained and traversing exceptionally beautiful forests filled with plenty of winding streams. Some of the mountain trails offer views of the surrounding mountains and farmlands; the best view is on Morrow Mountain, which is accessible by a road and has a paved parking lot at its peak. The Uwharrie National Forest (see pages 115 and 121) is 20 minutes to the east around Troy, North Carolina, with many more hiking and recreation opportunities. You can also explore the very cool (literally) underground trails of the Reed Gold Mine (see page 100), the site of historic ore veins, 40 minutes to the west in Midland, North Carolina.

Directions

From the Charlotte city center, merge onto US 74 East toward NC 27 and follow it for 3.8 miles. Merge onto NC 27 East via Exit 246 on the left and follow it for 38.2 miles. NC 27 East becomes NC 740 North. Follow NC 740 for 1.9 miles. Turn right onto Morrow Mountain Road/NC 1798. Continue to follow Morrow Mountain Road for 2.8 miles, where you reach the entrance to Morrow Mountain State Park. The trailhead is in the horse-trailer parking lot, the first turn to the right (south) after you enter the park. Follow the gravel road to the parking lot and park your vehicle.

14

Reed Gold Mine

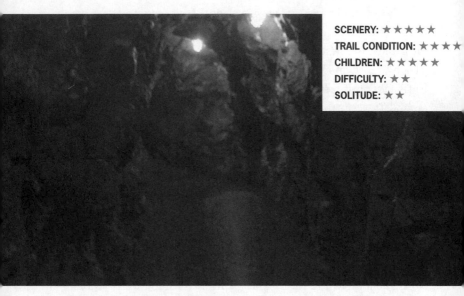

SCENERY: ★ ★ ★ ★ ★
TRAIL CONDITION: ★ ★ ★
CHILDREN: ★ ★ ★ ★ ★
DIFFICULTY: ★ ★
SOLITUDE: ★ ★

YOU MIGHT NOT FIND ANY RICHES, BUT YOU CAN DISCOVER SOME ADVENTURE WHEN YOU JOURNEY INTO THE COOL, DARK UNDERGROUND SHAFTS OF THE REED GOLD MINE.

GPS TRAILHEAD COORDINATES: N35° 17.102' W80° 27.934'

DISTANCE & CONFIGURATION: 0.9-mile loop

HIKING TIME: 2 hours

HIGHLIGHTS: Reed Gold Mine, Morgan Shaft, Stamp Mill, Little Meadow Creek, mine site, and museum

ELEVATION: 538' at the trailhead to 601'

ACCESS: Tuesday–Saturday, 9 a.m.–5 p.m.

MAPS: At the Reed Gold Mine Museum and Visitor's Center and **nchistoricsites.org/reed**

FACILITIES: Museum, restroom, and water fountains

WHEELCHAIR ACCESS: Only the museum

COMMENTS: Allow extra time for this trail—it's very interesting, and the underground self-guided tour really captures the imagination.

CONTACTS: (704) 721-4653; **nchistoricsites.org/reed**

Overview

Explore the historic site of the old Reed Gold Mine on this self-guided tour of the now-defunct mining operation. The highlight of the trail is near the start of your hike. You reach a large wooden door built into a hillside and descend belowground to explore underground mine shafts and routes of the mine. You don't need flashlights or a miner's cap. It's well lit throughout the underground portion of the trail and nice and cool down in the mine, making it a great trail during the peak heat of a Charlotte summer. Interpretive plaques throughout the above- and belowground trails provide a great explanation of everything you will be seeing, from mine shafts, mining tools, a stamp mill, and the other natural features on the route. This trail is great for everyone, including kids. If you only get a chance to do a handful of the trails in this book, I highly encourage you to explore the Reed Gold Mine.

Route Details

The trailhead is in front of the visitor center at the wide wooden bridge crossing Little Meadow Creek, where Conrad Reed, then only 12 years old, made the first documented discovery of gold in the United States. The boy found a 17-pound nugget in Little Meadow Creek. For a while the Reed family was even using it as a doorstop, until someone told them what it was. After the discovery, the first gold rush in the nation began, and the Reed Gold Mine started mining commercially in 1803.

The trail splits at the foot of the bridge. Stay left (northeast). Continue uphill 30 yards where the trail splits again. Stay left and head up the steep hill to a large wooden door at the entrance to the Reed Gold Mine. Enjoy the cold air underground in the mine. Take your time and explore the mine that ventures more than 55 feet underground. Interpretive plaques mark numbered stops along the subterranean portion of the trail. Each station has great information to explain what you're exploring, and the route is fairly self-explanatory.

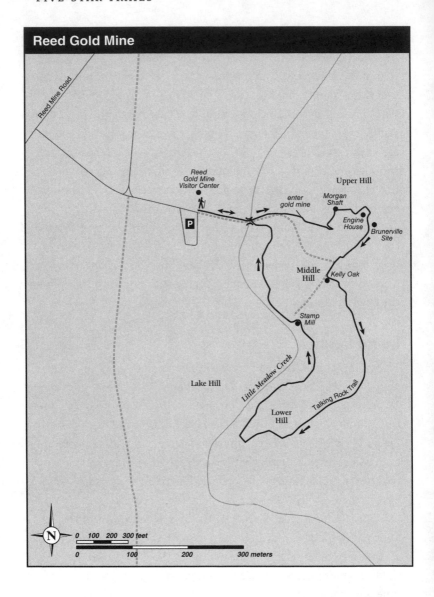

Reed Gold Mine

Reed Mine Road

Reed Gold Mine Visitor Center

P

enter gold mine

Morgan Shaft

Upper Hill

Engine House

Brunerville Site

Middle Hill

Kelly Oak

Stamp Mill

Little Meadow Creek

Lake Hill

Lower Hill

Talking Rock Trail

N

0 100 200 300 feet
0   100   200   300 meters

Meander through the well-lit mine and exit after a gradual ascent to the surface.

Behind the exit of the mine, to the north, is the Morgan shaft, which helped drill the mine and deliver tools and rock from the mine to the surface and back. Turn right (east) at the shaft and follow the concrete steps up to the foundation of the engine house. The route follows past an observation deck that gives you a nice aerial view of the engine house foundation and then leads along the north side of the foundation to a gravel road. Turn right (south) on the gravel road, passing by the Brunerville site (where the Reed Gold Company housed its workers) and the curious round Chilean stones used to extract gold from the mine.

Follow the gravel road to the split in the trail, and veer left toward the Kelly Oak, a tree more than 250 years old. Continue for 250 feet until you reach a junction at Kelly Oak. Turn left (southwest) toward Lower Hill and the Talking Rock Trail. This portion of the trail explores the aboveground operation processes and relics in more depth. You follow along dirt paths and boardwalks through a forest filled with what appear to be sinkholes but are actually old abandoned mine shafts; after 0.2 mile reach the mine site of Lower Hill. Continue around the looping Talking Rock Trail for another 0.2 mile until you reach the old, but restored, Stamp Mill, originally purchased in 1898. The trail actually enters the mill and follows the step up to the observation deck overlooking the mill. Then you head back down stairs leading to the Stamp Mill exit and onto the dirt path through the forest that parallels the creek bank. Follow the trail straight (north) for another 0.2 mile to the wide wooden bridge spanning Little Meadow Creek where you started, leading to the trailhead, parking lot, and visitor center.

Nearby Attractions

Uwharrie National Forest is 50 minutes to the east of Reed Gold Mine. There you will find hundreds of miles of hiking trails in the

50,640 acres of the Uwharrie, with some of the best trails in the Birkhead Wilderness Area to the northeast of Arrowhead campground. Also nearby is Morrow Mountain State Park, 45 minutes to the east. Morrow has more than 15 miles of hiking trails to explore. Climb challenging hills that offer nice views of the surrounding ridges and farmlands. The trails traverse exceptionally beautiful forests filled with plenty of winding streams.

Directions

Reed Gold Mine is 26 miles east of Charlotte, about 40 minutes from the Charlotte city center. From the Charlotte city center, take US 74 East 3.9 miles and merge onto NC 27 East via Exit 246 on the left; follow NC 27 for 18.6 miles. Turn left onto Reed Mine Road and follow it for 2.9 miles. Reed Gold Mine will be on the right. Drive into the Reed Gold Mine Park and park your vehicle in the parking lot in front of the museum and visitor center. Stop in at the museum to grab a map of the park and self-guided tour brochure.

15

Reedy Creek Nature Preserve: Dragonfly Pond Loop

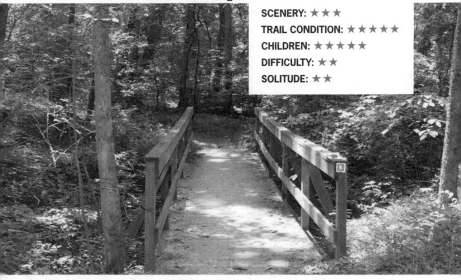

SCENERY: ★ ★ ★
TRAIL CONDITION: ★ ★ ★ ★ ★
CHILDREN: ★ ★ ★ ★ ★
DIFFICULTY: ★ ★
SOLITUDE: ★ ★

A WOODEN BRIDGE CROSSES REEDY CREEK.

GPS TRAILHEAD COORDINATES: N35° 15.695' W80° 43.122'

DISTANCE & CONFIGURATION: 1.5-mile loop

HIKING TIME: 1 hour

HIGHLIGHTS: Dragonfly Pond, historical building relics, fishing pier, volleyball court, and disc-golf course

ELEVATION: 757' at the trailhead to 662' at lowest point

ACCESS: Monday–Saturday, 9 a.m.–5 p.m.; Sunday, 1–5 p.m.

MAPS: At the Reedy Creek Nature Center, trailhead kiosks, park entrance, and **parkandrec .com/reedy**

FACILITIES: Restrooms, nature center, picnic shelters, Center for Biodiversity Studies, volleyball court, softball field, and fishing pier

WHEELCHAIR ACCESS: Yes, at the nature center facilities, restrooms, and some picnic shelters

COMMENTS: Dogs are allowed on leashes no longer than 6 feet in length. Swimming prohibited in ponds and other waterways.

CONTACTS: (704) 432-6459; **parkandrec.com/reedy**

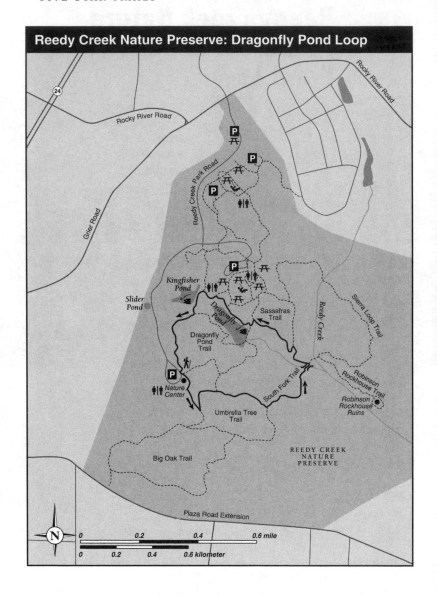

Reedy Creek Nature Preserve: Dragonfly Pond Loop

Overview

This short hike winds through the mature hardwood forests of Reedy Creek Nature Preserve. The trail traverses a variety of landscapes, including the magnolia-lined bank of Reedy Creek, open fields providing a perfect setting for an afternoon picnic, and the shore of Dragonfly Pond, where fishing is permitted. Ideal for kids, the trail begins near a playground and runs through a portion of a disc-golf course, past a volleyball court, and past several fishing piers. Come prepared and bring a rod and reel, a Frisbee, and volleyball, and use all the facilities along this beautiful trail.

Route Details

This region was one of the earliest European-occupied areas west of the Yadkin River. The favorable climate and rich soil for agriculture made the location popular with early settlers: along the trail you will encounter historical structural ruins and other signs of early inhabitation. You will also see an abundance of quartz and granite boulders dotting the landscape; settlers had to painstakingly remove

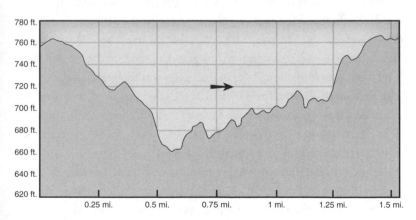

the boulders to prepare the land for farming. Along the trail, several clearings indicate where early settlers had planned homestead sites or farming fields.

Walk down the boardwalk to the nature center and follow the paved path past the playground and around the building to The Gathering Area, behind the nature center. Here you will find the trailhead to the Umbrella Tree Trail. A small kiosk holds trail maps as well as pocket-sized flora-and-fauna interpretive guides for this route. Walk down the gently sloping, gravel-and-sand, 5-foot-wide path into the forest. After 0.1 mile, you will pass a small field on your right.

At this small field you reach a junction with the Dragonfly Pond Trail. Stay on Umbrella Tree Trail by veering to the right or southeast. Along this portion of the trail you will pass many domed wigwamlike structures made from small saplings and branches. These interesting little forts were made during the preserve's programs for children. After 0.2 mile, turn left (east) onto South Fork Trail. Here the trail slopes gently downhill and narrows to a 3-foot-wide dirt track. The trail is well marked with red and white signs depicting a hiker with hiking stick. Continue for 0.3 mile until you cross a small bridge that crosses Reedy Creek. Then turn left (northwest) onto Sierra Loop Trail. This trail will follow along Reedy Creek's magnolia-lined bank to the left. Walk 0.1 mile and then turn left or south onto Sassafras Trail. The trail widens briefly with a gravel surface, and here you'll find a bench where you can take in the sights and sounds of the beautiful hardwood forest. If the bench is occupied, no need to worry; another one is waiting for you just 20 yards down the trail.

After 0.2 mile the trail leads into an open field on the shore of Dragonfly Pond, which is great for picnics, sunbathing, or a little Frisbee throwing. Here turn left or south onto Dragonfly Pond Trail. Follow Dragonfly Pond Trail along the pond's northern shore. An observation and fishing deck extends over the pond at several points along the trail, and on this section you will pass a sand-volleyball court and picnic shelters with barbecue grills. Behind the volleyball court is a red building with restrooms inside.

Continue for 0.3 mile and then turn left or south onto Kingfisher Pond Trail. This portion of the route passes through a section of the disc-golf course and runs along the shore of Kingfisher Pond. Walk 450 feet on the Kingfisher Pond Trail and then take a right or west to rejoin Dragonfly Pond Trail. The trail here passes a small enclosed area on the left that contains remnants of structures built by early inhabitants. Continue on Dragonfly Pond Trail until the trail exits into the nature center parking lot.

Nearby Attractions

The Reedy Creek Nature Center has exhibits featuring live native animals of the area and offers interpretive talks and programs for visitors. Outside the center are a bird-feeding station and butterfly garden. If you're interested in fishing any of the ponds in the preserve, check out a fishing pole and tackle for free here. Also in the preserve are the ruins of the Robinson Rockhouse, believed to have been built in 1790. The site was excavated by University of North Carolina at Charlotte archeologists and can be explored through an interpretive tour of the historical site.

Directions

From the Charlotte city center, follow I-85 North toward Greenville to Exit 45A. Merge onto East W. T. Harris Boulevard and follow it 3.3 miles. Turn left on Rocky River Road, and drive 0.5 mile. Turn left at the stoplight, continuing on Rocky River Road until you reach the entrance to the preserve, on the right. Follow the signs to the nature-center parking lot.

16

University of North Carolina at Charlotte Botanical Gardens

SCENERY: ★ ★ ★ ★ ★
TRAIL CONDITION: ★ ★ ★ ★ ★
CHILDREN: ★ ★ ★ ★ ★
DIFFICULTY: ★ ★
SOLITUDE: ★ ★

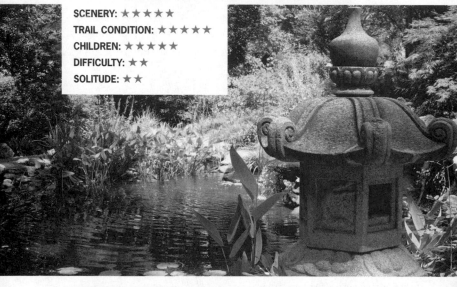

A VIEW OF THE JAPANESE GARDEN FROM THE EDGE OF THE POND

GPS TRAILHEAD COORDINATES: N35° 18.464' W80° 43.758'

DISTANCE & CONFIGURATION: 0.3-mile balloon

HIKING TIME: 1 hour

HIGHLIGHTS: Greenhouse, gardens, gazebo, and pond

ELEVATION: 704' at the trailhead to 672' at lowest point

ACCESS: Daily, sunrise–sunset

MAPS: At trailhead kiosk, campus visitor center, and the greenhouse across from the trailhead

FACILITIES: Restrooms in nearby greenhouse

WHEELCHAIR ACCESS: None

COMMENTS: During regular school hours, the main trail leading to the botanical gardens can be congested with students using the trail to get to and from class, but the actual botanical gardens usually aren't very crowded. The parking garages on campus accept only cash.

CONTACTS: (704) 687-0720; **gardens.uncc.edu**

Overview

These beautiful botanical gardens, on the east side of the University of North Carolina (UNC) at Charlotte campus, are definitely worth a visit. Each section of the garden is unique in design and captures the essence of gardening in various parts of the world as part of the international theme. Apart from the wonderful flora that can be explored on the grounds, an exceptional amount of impressive architectural design and artful craftsmanship have gone into the garden's many bridges, art displays, gazebos, and trellises. The trail begins near UNC's McMillan Greenhouse, where you can peek in and check out all the exotic plants the professors are cultivating. Then head onto the trail and into the Susie Harwood Garden for a pleasant walk that feels more like an adventure through gardens of the world. This trail is highly recommended for children.

Route Details

Directly across the main road from the greenhouse is a large gravel trail. It looks more like a road, as it is more than 12 feet wide and leads down a fairly steep hill to the entrance of the Susie Harwood Garden on your left (northwest). At the kiosk you can conveniently pick up a map to the garden. They even offer a laminated map if you are here when it is raining. Standing at the kiosk and looking down the trail, turn left (northeast) up the gravel-covered steps and into the Susie Harwood Garden. The setting is beautifully landscaped, and the trees, plants, and shrubs are all very well described by interpretive plaques. Frequent benches provide ample spots to sit and take in the sights and sounds of the garden.

Stay on the main trail and follow the path, crossing over a shallow creek via a small bridge with red metal handrails. At the end of the bridge, turn left (northwest) and follow the trail uphill to the hummingbird and butterfly garden. The artfully designed rock garden is on your left, and here you can take a short side trail to explore it. Just around the bend on your right, you pass a tall wooden arbor,

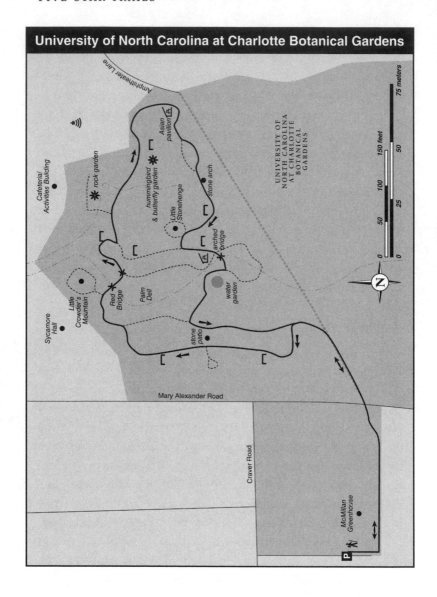

University of North Carolina at Charlotte Botanical Gardens

the centerpiece of the hummingbird and butterfly garden. Follow the trail, continuing to climb uphill, to a beautiful pavilion constructed in a Japanese architectural style that marks the entrance to the Asian garden. Follow the stone path around to the left and through the thought-provoking circular stone arch, my personal favorite part of the garden. Something about the arch somehow forces me to recognize and reflect on where I am and what I am experiencing in the current moment.

Continue to follow the path downhill and down the stone steps to the red Asian-style gazebo. A wonderfully landscaped pond with a tranquil fountain sits just in front of the gazebo, making this the perfect place to stop for a rest or to have lunch. The elevated gazebo provides a wonderful view of the pond and the garden that surrounds it. To the south of the gazebo, cross the arched bridge that spans the main creek and turn right (west) to follow the trail running in front of the pond. Once you reach the main trail again, turn left (east) to return to the trailhead at the base of the steep hill and the exit toward the greenhouse.

Nearby Attractions

Unless you want to visit the UNC library while you're on campus, there isn't a whole lot for visitors to do. In the greater university area of Charlotte, you can explore more trails at nearby Reedy Creek Nature Preserve (see page 105), just 3 miles southeast of campus. Right around campus are several strip malls with restaurants and retail stores. An exceptional variety of international cuisine and pizza joints caters to the college crowd. Of note is The Flying Saucer Emporium, which serves tasty hot dogs and burgers and offers a large variety of beers on tap; it's always a favorite with students. For something a little more international, try the Casablanca Café, the Thai House, or Amalfi Pasta and Pizza. The strip mall just across University City Boulevard also has a Harris Teeter grocery store—a good place to stop for snacks and drinks before your garden walk. The

Marriott Courtyard and the Hilton near the university are recommended hotels.

Directions

Uptown Charlotte is about 20 minutes from the university. From the Charlotte city center, take I-277 South and follow it for 0.6 mile. Merge onto I-77 North/US 21 North via Exit 1C toward Statesville and follow it for 3.4 miles. Merge onto I-85 North via Exit 13A toward Greensboro and follow it for 4.2 miles. Merge onto US 29–Bypass North via Exit 42 toward US 29/NC 49 and follow it for 1.0 mile. Stay straight to go onto North Tryon Street/US 29 North/NC 49 North and follow it for 2.5 miles. Continue to follow NC 49 North to 9201 University City Boulevard and the campus main entrance, on the left. Drive into the university's main entrance off University City Boulevard/NC 49. Take the first exit to the right in the roundabout, and follow the signs to the greenhouse. Parking at the greenhouse is usually full. If the greenhouse parking is all taken, there are two different visitor parking garages, back the way you came in, that charge $1 per 30 minutes. *Note:* The parking garages on campus are cash-only, so come prepared.

17

Uwharrie National Forest: Badin Lake Trail

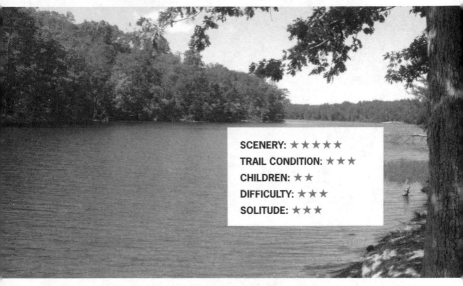

SCENERY: ★ ★ ★ ★ ★
TRAIL CONDITION: ★ ★ ★
CHILDREN: ★ ★
DIFFICULTY: ★ ★ ★
SOLITUDE: ★ ★ ★

VIEWS OF BADIN LAKE ABOUND ALONG THIS UWHARRIE NATIONAL FOREST TRAIL.

GPS TRAILHEAD COORDINATES: N35° 26.351' W80° 04.346'

DISTANCE & CONFIGURATION: 5.5-mile loop

HIKING TIME: 3.5 hours

HIGHLIGHTS: Badin Lake, Arrowhead Campground, picnic facilities, and boat launch

ELEVATION: 582' at the trailhead to 650' to 504' at the lowest point

ACCESS: Daily, 7 a.m.–9 p.m.; Arrowhead campsites $15 per night

MAPS: At the U.S. Forest Service office in Troy, North Carolina; the Arrowhead Campground host; and **fs.usda.gov/nfsnc**

FACILITIES: Restrooms, showers at campground, water spigots, picnic pavilions, and boat launch

WHEELCHAIR ACCESS: None

COMMENTS: This trail follows alongside Badin Lake for some distance. During the summer months, when the bugs and mosquitoes are active, it's a good idea to bring insect repellent along. The trail follows very close to the lakeshore at times, and along here you're likely to find snakes, particularly venomous

Uwharrie National Forest: Badin Lake Trail

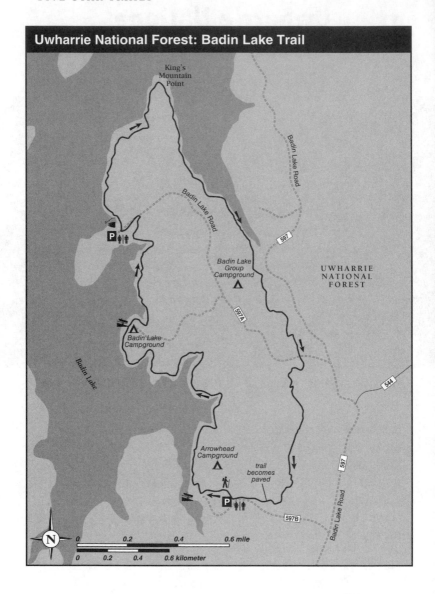

King's
Mountain
Point

Badin Lake Road

597

Badin Lake Road

UWHARRIE
NATIONAL
FOREST

Badin Lake
Group
Campground

P

597A

Badin Lake
Campground

Badin Lake

544

Arrowhead
Campground

trail
becomes
paved

597

P

597B

Badin Lake Road

N

| 0 | | 0.2 | | 0.4 | | 0.6 mile |

| 0 | 0.2 | 0.4 | 0.6 kilometer |

water moccasins, so keep your eyes open while hiking this route. This trail is shared with bikers, so be conscious of them and give them the right-of-way. Hunting is permitted in the Uwharrie National Forest. Hunting seasons run September–December. Be sure to hike with caution, and consider wearing orange vests or other bright clothing to ensure that you are visible to hunters during the hunting seasons.

CONTACTS: (910) 576-6391; **fs.usda.gov/nfsnc**

Overview

The Badin Lake Trail starts from the Arrowhead Campground on a spur trail near the bathhouse. Hike down to the Arrowhead Campground boat launch and explore the shore of Badin Lake and the surrounding forest. The hike is mostly level and pretty well marked. At times the trail traverses over exposed rock areas, so it's a good idea to wear some good hiking shoes or tennis shoes that have adequate grip for this trail. Along the way you'll find plenty of exceptional fishing spots, a sandy shoreline, and rocky resting spots with fantastic views of the lake.

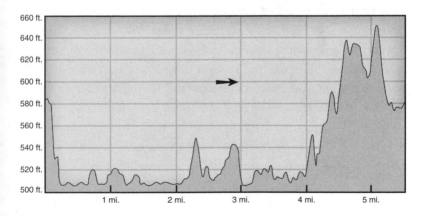

Route Details

From your parking spot, walk toward the restrooms and follow the paved road as it veers left. Turn left (west) onto the paved trail at the trailhead, marked with a sign that reads HIKERS AND BIKERS ONLY. This is a spur trail that leads to the Arrowhead Trail, which circles the campground. After 20 yards the trail splits. Veer right toward the lake. After 40 yards you reach another junction. Turn left (west) onto the white-blazed Badin Lake Trail. The 4-foot-wide dirt path leads to a series of steps that lead downhill to the boat launch. Once you reach the parking lot, white arrows painted on the pavement to the right will direct you around the parking lot and back onto the trail.

The trail follows along the lakeshore. This section is easy to follow and well marked, although the trail gets slightly rocky in places. You pass several nice open clearings along the lakeshore that make for good picnic or resting spots. From the boat launch you walk 1.3 miles until you pass through the Badin Lake Campground, with restrooms, picnic tables, and drinking water spigots as well as water fountains. The trail continues along the lake and passes directly in front of several campsites and then passes in front of a small boat launch ramp. After 0.9 mile from Badin Lake Campground you reach the parking lot for the King's Mountain Point recreation area. A wooden dock and a fishing pier extend into Lake Badin. There are more restrooms here as well. This section of the trail is very poorly marked and can be very confusing. When you come out into the parking lot, look across to the other side, where you will see small brown signs that are way too small to make navigating the trail easy, and enter back into the forest. Follow the trail to King's Mountain Point. A beautiful campsite in a shaded clearing features a stone fire ring and excellent views of the lake. From the parking lot for King's Mountain Recreation Area, it's 0.9 mile to King's Mountain Point.

As you reach the end of the lake, you see some very nice homes on the opposite side of the water with interesting pier designs. Pass through the small primitive group camp and behind a privately owned lot of land. The trail enters into the forest and meanders through the forest along the creek. After 1.3 miles from King's Mountain Point, you cross a gravel road, 597-A. Eighty yards after crossing the gravel road, the trail briefly joins the green-blazed Josh Trail and then splits to the left, where the white blazes and the Badin Lake Trail continue. The path becomes thinner and the forest exceptionally dense before the trail crosses the green-blazed Lake Trail. Signs note that at this point you are 0.5 mile from Arrowhead Campground. After 80 more yards the trail crosses 597-B, a gravel road. After 0.5 mile more the trail becomes paved as it gets close to the campground. Shortly after the trail becomes paved, the path splits. Veer to the left (west) and, after 40 yards, cross the campground's main paved road to continue on the Arrowhead Trail. The trail curves around tent campsites and then returns to the parking lot and trailhead. There are many different

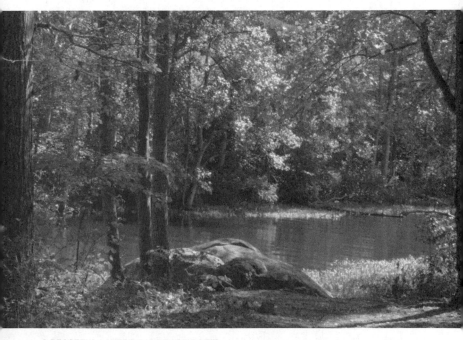

A PEACEFUL LAKESIDE VANTAGE POINT

paths that you can take during this last section that will lead you back to the trailhead and parking lot. This is the most direct way to get back to where you started your hike.

Nearby Attractions

The Arrowhead Campground has 50 sites, each with electricity, a picnic table, and a tent pad. The campground also offers good hot showers in the bathhouse and a boat ramp. There are literally hundreds of miles of hiking trails in the 50,640 acres of the Uwharrie, with some of the best in the Birkhead Wilderness Area (see next profile) to the northeast of Arrowhead Campground. Morrow Mountain State Park (see pages 90 and 95), 20 minutes to the west of Uwharrie, has more than 15 miles of hiking trails to explore; most of them are more demanding than the trails you find in the Uwharrie, with challenging hills that offer nice views of the surrounding ridges and farmlands and exceptionally beautiful forests filled with plenty of winding streams. Reed Gold Mine (see page 100) is 45 minutes to the southwest near Midland, North Carolina.

Directions

From NC 109 North in Troy, go to Mullinix Road just past Macedonia Church. Turn left onto Mullinix and continue past Horse Camp. Turn right on FR 544 and follow it for 1.8 miles; then turn left on FR 597 and follow it for 0.6 mile. Turn right on FR 597B to the entrance of the campground. Park at the parking lot near the bathhouse on the western side of the campground, near campsite 42.

18

Uwharrie National Forest: Birkhead Mountains Wilderness Trail

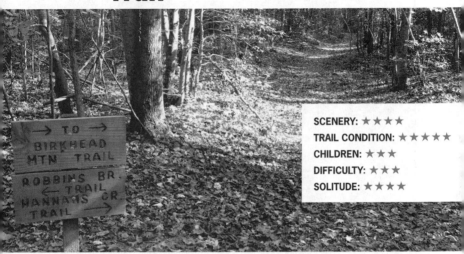

SCENERY: ★ ★ ★ ★
TRAIL CONDITION: ★ ★ ★ ★ ★
CHILDREN: ★ ★ ★
DIFFICULTY: ★ ★ ★
SOLITUDE: ★ ★ ★ ★

IF IT'S SOLITUDE YOU SEEK, HEAD TO THE BIRKHEAD MOUNTAINS WILDERNESS TRAIL.

GPS TRAILHEAD COORDINATES: N35° 35.433' W79° 56.898'

DISTANCE & CONFIGURATION: 6.7-mile balloon

HIKING TIME: 4 hours

HIGHLIGHTS: Birkhead Mountain, Robbins Branch Creek, and Hannah's Creek

ELEVATION: 589' at the trailhead to 909'

ACCESS: Daily, 7 a.m.–9 p.m.; Arrowhead campsites $15 per night

MAPS: At the U.S. Forest Service office in Troy, North Carolina, and **tinyurl.com/birkheadmap**

FACILITIES: None

WHEELCHAIR ACCESS: None

COMMENTS: There are no maps at the trailhead and no water or other facilities in the forest, so come prepared. Hunting is permitted in the Uwharrie National Forest (seasons run September–December). Be sure to hike with caution, and consider wearing orange vests or other bright clothing to ensure that you are visible to hunters during the hunting seasons.

CONTACTS: (910) 576-6391; **fs.usda.gov/nfsnc**

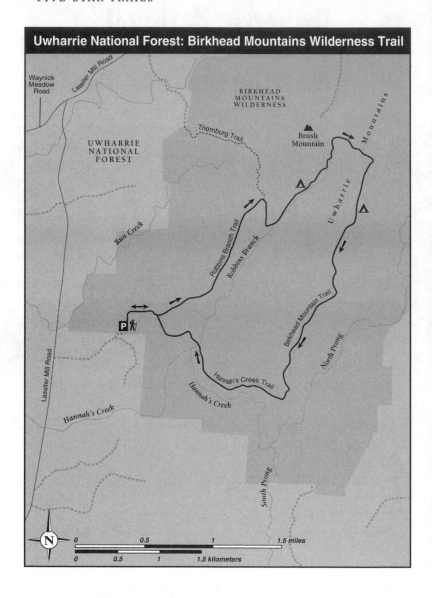

Uwharrie National Forest: Birkhead Mountains Wilderness Trail

Waynick Meadow Road

Lassiter Mill Road

BIRKHEAD MOUNTAINS WILDERNESS

Thornburg Trail

Brush Mountain

Uwharrie Mountains

UWHARRIE NATIONAL FOREST

Run Creek

Robbins Branch Trail

Robbins Branch

Birkhead Mountain Trail

North Prong

Lassiter Mill Road

P

Hannah's Creek Trail

Hannah's Creek

Hannah's Creek

South Prong

N

0   0.5   1   1.5 miles

0   0.5   1   1.5 kilometers

Overview

This long loop through the heart of the Birkhead Wilderness combines three trails—the Robbins Branch Trail, Hannah's Creek Trail, and the Birkhead Mountain Trail—to create a challenging loop from the trailhead at the end of Robbins Branch Road. The long trail traverses a series of challenging hills and climbs up to the peak of Birkhead Mountain almost 1,000 feet high. You won't get spectacular views here as you would in South Mountains State Park and along other trails west of Charlotte, but the trail does follow and cross several nice creeks. The forest in this area is mature and beautiful, and the wilderness designation keeps it from being overused by other recreationists, making it a great place for hiking, birding, and wildlife viewing. The trail and the wilderness it's in are real hidden gems to the east of Charlotte. The best camping is 20 minutes to the southwest at Arrowhead Campground, just outside the town of Uwharrie.

Route Details

You won't find any maps at the trailhead—you'll need to pick them up at the ranger station in Troy before you head out to the wilderness,

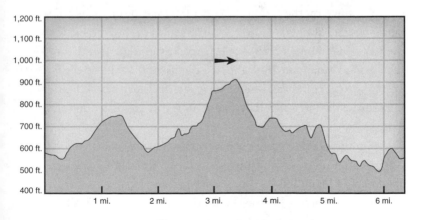

or go to the website mentioned previously and print out maps before you go. There isn't even a sign or kiosk at the trailhead that marks the trail as Robbins Branch Trail. Only a couple of really large boulders and sliced-through fallen pine trees mark the trailhead, where a 3-foot-wide dirt path leads into the forest. Continue on the Robbins Branch Trail, blazed with white rectangles, for 0.3 mile until you reach a split in the trail. Hannah's Creek Trail splits to the right (southeast). Stay left (northeast) and continue on the Robbins Branch Trail. Along this section, the forest becomes noticeably younger, thicker, and denser, with a thicket of closely growing spindly oaks and pines.

After 1.8 miles, during which distance you climb over a large hill and begin to ascend your second, the trail splits again. To the left (north) is the Thornburg Trailhead. Stay to the right (south) and continue following the Robbins Branch Trail. Along this section, the trail crosses Robbins Branch Creek several times via wooden footbridges, and after 0.6 mile you reach a campsite along the creek. This section of the trail can be a bit confusing, as it is not very well marked. Keep your eye out for the white blazes on the trees. The trail runs parallel to the creek, so if you walk along the creek bank, you'll eventually spot a white blaze on a tree after 20–30 yards or so.

Continue on the trail for another 0.9 mile, during which distance you climb over two more hills, until you reach the junction with the Birkhead Mountain Trail. At the junction, turn right (south) onto the Birkhead Mountain Trail. The trail climbs for 0.1 mile up the last hill to the top of Birkhead Mountain, where you reach a backcountry campsite marked by a sign that reads CAMP 5. It's a small camp with a large stone fire pit.

Continue hiking along the Birkhead Mountain Trail for another 0.4 mile until you reach the junction with the Hannah's Creek Trail. The Birkhead Mountain Trail continues straight and ends at Strieby Church Road. Turn right (west) onto the Hannah's Creek Trail and continue toward the Robbins Branch Trailhead. The trail is easy to follow from this point. You have one more large hill to climb, and then the trail gradually descends over a series of small hills for 1.4

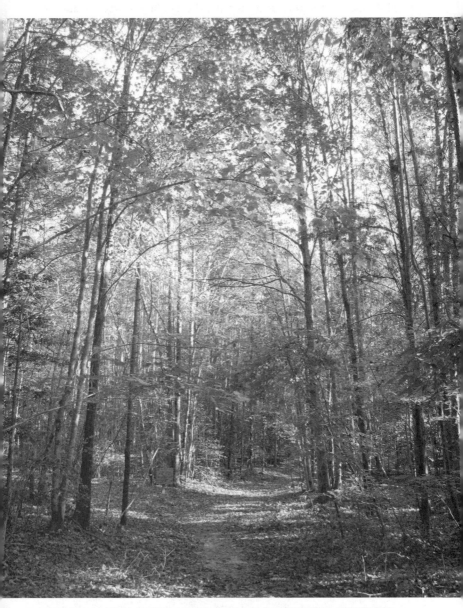

MORE THAN 6 MILES OF TRAILS SPAN THE 5,160-ACRE BIRKHEAD WILDERNESS.

miles back to the intersection with the Robbins Branch Trailhead. Once you reach the Robbins Branch Trail, stay straight (northwest) for 0.3 mile back to the trailhead, parking lot, and end of the Robbins Branch Trail.

Nearby Attractions

Arrowhead Campground is 15 miles southwest of the Birkhead Wilderness. There are literally hundreds of miles of hiking trails in the 50,640 acres of the Uwharrie National Forest, with some of them in the Birkhead Wilderness and the area around Arrowhead Campground (see page 115). The campground has 50 sites, each with electricity, a picnic table, and a tent pad. The campground also offers good hot showers in the bathhouse and a boat ramp. Morrow Mountain State Park (see pages 90 and 95), 20 minutes to the west of Uwharrie, has more than 15 miles of hiking trails to explore; most of them are more demanding than the trails you find in the Uwharrie, with challenging hills that offer nice views of the surrounding ridges and farmlands and exceptionally beautiful forests filled with plenty of winding streams. Reed Gold Mine (see page 100) is 45 minutes to the southwest near Midland, North Carolina.

Directions

First things first: the signage along the road going to this trail is bad, very bad—definitely the worst road signage of any of the trails in this book—but don't let that discourage you. Stay focused, keeping your eyes peeled and sticking to the directions to find the trail. It's easy enough to get to Lassiter Mill Road, but the hard part is finding Robbins Branch Road. The best way to find it is to look for a small brown sign (on the western side of Lassiter Mill Road) that has an arrow pointing to the gravel and moderately steep Robbins Branch Road and reads BIRKHEAD WILDERNESS. The gravel road leads uphill for 0.7 mile and dead-ends at the trailhead to the Robbins Branch Trail.

From Troy take NC 109 north to the town of Uwharrie. Turn right on Ophir Road and follow it for 7.1 miles. Ophir Road becomes Burney Mill Road. Follow Burney Mill Road for 0.9 mile. Turn right onto Lassiter Mill Road and follow it for 2.4 miles. Turn right onto the unmarked Robbins Branch Road, where a brown sign marks the road as leading to the Birkhead Wilderness. Follow up the gravel and steep Robbins Branch Road for 0.7 mile until you reach a dead-end, a parking lot, and the Robbins Branch Trailhead.

South of Charlotte (Hikes 19–24)

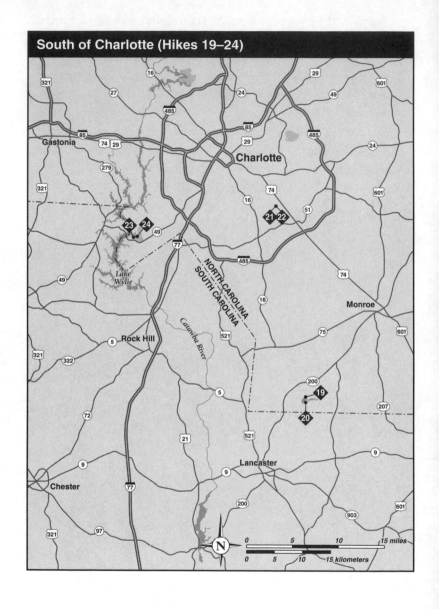

South of Charlotte

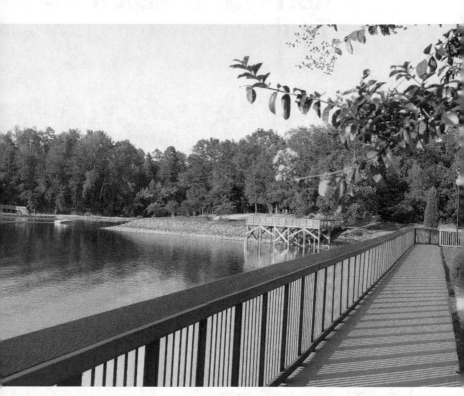

A WALKWAY HUGS THE SHORE OF LAKE WYLIE IN THE McDOWELL NATURE PRESERVE.

19 **Cane Creek Park: Northern Red Loop Trail**

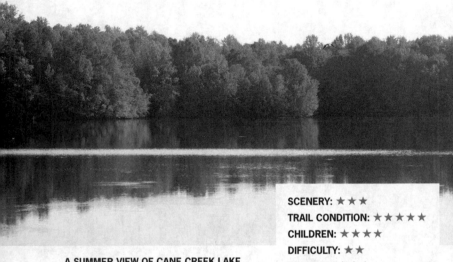

SCENERY: ★ ★ ★
TRAIL CONDITION: ★ ★ ★ ★ ★
CHILDREN: ★ ★ ★ ★
DIFFICULTY: ★ ★
SOLITUDE: ★ ★ ★

A SUMMER VIEW OF CANE CREEK LAKE

GPS TRAILHEAD COORDINATES: N34° 50.609' W80° 41.160'

DISTANCE & CONFIGURATION: 3.4-mile loop

HIKING TIME: 2.5 hours

HIGHLIGHTS: Cane Creek Lake, boat launch, Cane Creek, forest, recreation fields, and climbing wall

ELEVATION: 618' at the trailhead to 554' at lowest point

ACCESS: Daily, 7 a.m.–7 p.m.; campsites are $15–$20

MAPS: At the park visitor center and **co.union.nc.us**

FACILITIES: Restrooms, water fountains, campground, miniature golf, climbing wall, amphitheater, rental boats, picnic facilities, fishing rentals, and workout stations

WHEELCHAIR ACCESS: Some of the trails in the park are wheelchair-accessible. However, this trail is not.

COMMENTS: Sections of this loop trail are shared with horses. Give horses the right-of-way. The trails marked with yellow blazes are hiker-only.

CONTACTS: (704) 843-3919; **co.union.nc.us**

Overview

The Red Loop hike starts in the northern portion of Cane Creek Park and is more than 3 miles long but has little elevation. It's an easy hike through mostly forested terrain. A good hike for older kids who can handle the 3-mile trek, the trail passes a climbing wall station, soccer field, and Cane Creek Lake. Several spur trails lead to nice picnic pavilions, and with all of the recreation opportunities along the route, it's easy enough to make a whole day of the hike.

Route Details

After parking, walk north past the entrance station and back up the park's main paved road to the trailhead marked by a brown sign. The trail has two entrances. One of the trails goes to the ball field. Take the 4-foot-wide dirt trail on the left, marked LOOP TRAIL and blazed with red squares.

The trail is shared with horses, so be sure to give them the right-of-way if you encounter them. The path runs alongside the road and is very easy to follow. It descends to a soccer field, which can be seen through the trees to the right (south). After 0.1 mile you pass the Orange Trail, on your right. Continue straight on the Red Loop Trail. Continue for an additional 0.1 mile until the trail splits in two directions. To the right, the Blue Trail, blazed with blue markers, leads to the southern section of the Red Loop Trail. Stay left (northeast) on the Red Loop Trail. It's common to see deer on this trail, so keep your eyes open and you might catch a glimpse. After 0.4 mile from the junction with the Blue Trail, the Red Loop Trail gets close to the road before veering off to the right (south) and leaving the road behind. From here the path gradually descends for 0.8 mile down to the lake, passing under power lines and the clearing they create. Once the trail reaches the lake, it veers to the right (southwest) and begins to follow along the lakeshore for 0.2 mile. During this section the trail goes over several small hills and crosses a creek. After leaving the lake, the Red Loop Trail intersects

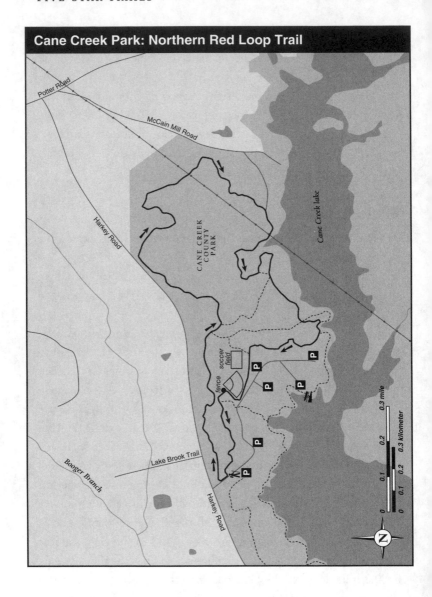

Cane Creek Park: Northern Red Loop Trail

with the Blue Trail. Stay left (west) on the Red Loop Trail, which rejoins the lakeshore.

Along this next section of the Red Loop Trail, which follows along the shore of Badin Lake, spurs lead to the Blue, Orange, and Yellow trails. Stay straight on the Red Loop Trail. After 0.4 mile, the Red Loop Trail leaves the lake behind and passes restrooms and a recreation field on the left (west). The trail continues 0.3 mile and then takes a sharp turn to the left (west). From here the Red Loop Trail crosses a large soccer field. Walk for 0.2 mile, passing the baseball field, climbing wall, and the exercise area with pull-up bars and sit-up benches. In this area there are also picnic pavilions, restrooms, water fountains, a volleyball field, and smaller picnic areas with grills. The trail can be a bit confusing at this point. Follow the thin dirt path that runs along the front of the baseball field's chain-link fence. Once you reach the corner of the ball field, the trail wraps around the side of the ball field and reaches a wooden fence. Turn sharply left (west) by the baseball field dugout to reenter the forest. Interpretive plaques lining the trail on this next section identify and describe the trees and plants along the way. Continue 0.3 mile until you reach the trailhead at the park's main paved road. The parking lot and the park entrance station are to your left (west).

Nearby Attractions

More than 14 miles of trails crisscross Cane Creek Park. The southern section of the park also has a campground and additional recreation facilities. The campground, on the shore of Cane Creek Lake, has a camp store, hot showers, picnic facilities, mini golf, and restrooms. The town of Rock Hill is just a little more than 30 minutes to the west, and Charlotte is only 45 minutes to the north.

Directions

From the Charlotte city center, take I-277 South/US 74 West, and follow it for 0.8 mile. Merge onto I-77 South/US 21 South via exit 1B toward Columbia and follow it for 7 miles. Merge onto I-485 East via Exit 2 toward Martin/Pineville and follow it for 11.5 miles. Take the NC 16/Providence Road exit, Exit 57, toward Weddington and follow it for 0.3 mile. Turn right onto Providence Road South/NC 16 and follow it for 9.8 miles. Turn left onto East South Main Street/NC 75/Providence Road South/Waxhaw Highway. Continue on Providence Road South and follow it for 2.1 miles. Turn right to stay on Providence Road South and follow it for 5 miles. Turn left onto Harkey Road and follow it for 1.1 miles. The park is on the right. Park in the parking lot just past the entrance station to the northern section of Cane Creek Park. The southern section contains the campground, and the northern section is considered the day-use area.

20 **Cane Creek Park:
Southern Trails**

SCENERY: ★ ★ ★
TRAIL CONDITION: ★ ★ ★ ★ ★
CHILDREN: ★ ★ ★ ★
DIFFICULTY: ★ ★
SOLITUDE: ★ ★ ★

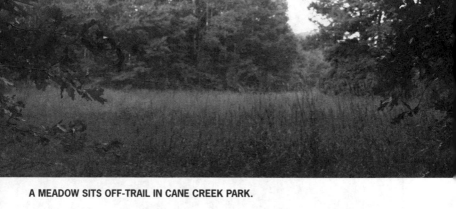

A MEADOW SITS OFF-TRAIL IN CANE CREEK PARK.

GPS TRAILHEAD COORDINATES: N34° 50.077' W80° 41.148'

DISTANCE & CONFIGURATION: 3.6-mile balloon

HIKING TIME: 3 hours

HIGHLIGHTS: Cane Creek Lake, Cane Creek, forest, meadows, and picnic facilities

ELEVATION: 558' at the trailhead to 620'

ACCESS: Daily, 7 a.m.–7 p.m.; campsites are $15–$20

MAPS: At the park visitor center and **co.union.nc.us**

FACILITIES: Water fountains, campground, miniature golf, rental boats, picnic facilities, and
fishing rentals

WHEELCHAIR ACCESS: Some of the trails in the park are wheelchair-accessible. However,
this trail is not.

COMMENTS: Sections of this loop trail are shared with horses. Give horses the right-of-
way. The trails marked with yellow blazes are hiker-only.

CONTACTS: (704) 843-3919; **co.union.nc.us**

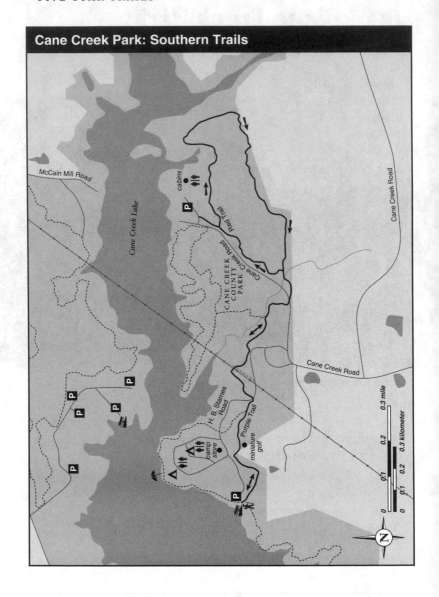

Cane Creek Park: Southern Trails

Overview

Starting from the southern section of Cane Creek Park, this trail departs from the primitive-camping parking lot on the shore of Cane Creek Lake. The route combines two popular trails in the park to create a simple balloon hike. Hike along the shore of Cane Creek Lake before exploring the surrounding forest. An extensive picnic-pavilion development about halfway through the hike makes for a well-positioned resting point.

Route Details

The trailhead is on the southern end of the parking lot, at the opposite side of the parking spaces. The trail almost immediately splits. Turn left (east) and continue on the Purple Trail, which runs behind the campsites, toward the camp store and the entrance of the park. The trail climbs gently uphill and winds through the forest away from the lake. Once you reach the camp store, avoid the road along the fence and stay on the well-marked trail that runs behind the mini golf course. The path slowly moves uphill and passes a small but pleasant meadow on the right (southwest), where you reach a junction with the Yellow Trail. Stay straight (south) on the Purple Trail, and after 40 yards cross the main road.

The path descends downhill to a shallow creek and crosses a very small wooden footbridge. After 500 feet more, the trail passes under power lines, through a small campground, and across a gravel road. After another 300 feet, the trail descends to Cane Creek. Here, ferns and other water-loving plants line the creek edge. The soil in this section is sandy and covered in moss in some places, and boulders and rocks have been exposed around the edge of the creek. The trail follows along the pleasant creek for 0.6 mile until you reach the junction with the Blue Trail. Stay straight (southwest) on the Purple Trail. Continue for another 0.2 mile, crossing several small streams, until the trail intersects with the Red Trail. Turn left (west) onto the Red Trail, walking toward the group campsites and cabins. After 0.5

mile you reach the cabins and group campsites. Here the trail gets rather confusing—if you don't pay attention, you'll easily take the spur trail that leads to the paved road and the cabins. Instead of doing this, turn right (west) and follow the Red Trail behind the cabins. Stay behind the cabins on the Red Trail. Cross a gravel road and then walk through two meadows, which make a good spot for a picnic with tables on the left side of the trail. These meadows can be a bit confusing, too, but they're kept mowed to make it easier to follow the trail. And if you look hard enough, you can spot a few red blazes on trees on the other side of the meadows.

Continue on the trail through the forest. This section is very easy to follow. The trail simply loops back around for 1.1 miles until you reach the Purple Trail again. Once you reach the junction, follow the Purple Trail back to the primitive campground and boat launch where you started. The Purple Trail intersects the Blue and Yellow trails, but stay on the Purple Trail, which will take you back to the parking lot and the trailhead where you started.

Nearby Attractions

More than 14 miles of trails cover Cane Creek Park. The southern section of the park also has a campground and more recreation facilities. The campground, on the shore of Cane Creek Lake, has a store, hot showers, picnic facilities, mini golf, and restrooms. The town of Rock Hill is just a little more than 30 minutes to the west, and Charlotte is only 45 minutes to the north.

Directions

From the Charlotte city center, take I-277 South/US 74 West and follow it for 0.8 mile. Merge onto I-77 South/US 21 South via Exit 1B toward Columbia and follow it for 7 miles. Merge onto I-485 East via Exit 2 toward Martin/Pineville and follow it for 11.5 miles. Take the NC 16/Providence Road exit, Exit 57, toward Weddington and follow it for 0.3 mile. Turn right onto Providence Road South/NC 16 and follow it for 9.8 miles. Turn left onto East South Main Street/NC 75/ Providence Road South/Waxhaw Highway. Continue on Providence Road South and follow it for 2.1 miles. Turn right to stay on Providence Road South and follow it for 5 miles. Turn left onto Harkey Road and follow it for 1.1 miles. The park is on the right. Park at the wilderness-camping and boat-launch parking lot, in the southern part of Cane Creek Park.

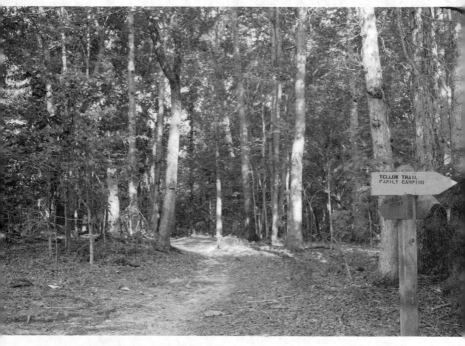

PICK YOUR PATH AND FOLLOW THE SIGNS.

McAlpine Creek
Greenway Loop

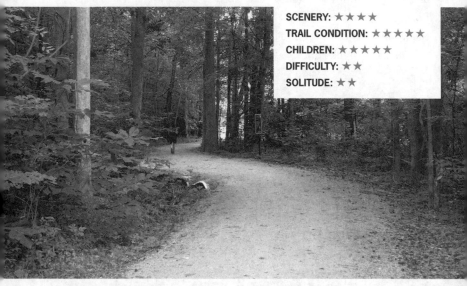

SCENERY: ★ ★ ★ ★
TRAIL CONDITION: ★ ★ ★ ★ ★
CHILDREN: ★ ★ ★ ★ ★
DIFFICULTY: ★ ★
SOLITUDE: ★ ★

THIS GRAVEL LOOP ALONG THE McALPINE CREEK GREENWAY IS A POPULAR WALKING ROUTE FOR RESIDENTS OF SOUTH CHARLOTTE.

GPS TRAILHEAD COORDINATES: N35° 9.013' W80° 44.659'

DISTANCE & CONFIGURATION: 1.9-mile figure eight

HIKING TIME: 3 hours

HIGHLIGHTS: Soccer fields, pond, open-air auditorium, dog park, 5k cross-country trail, and owl-nesting site

ELEVATION: 585' at the trailhead to 567' at lowest point

ACCESS: Daily, sunrise–sunset

MAPS: At Charlotte Visitor Info Center, trailhead kiosks, and **parkandrec.com**

FACILITIES: Restrooms and water fountains

WHEELCHAIR ACCESS: Yes, on paved paths around pond and to restrooms.

COMMENTS: Dogs are allowed on leashes 6 feet or shorter; you'll share the trail with runners, walkers, and bikers.

CONTACTS: (704) 432-1570; **parkandrec.com**

Overview

This route begins at McAlpine Creek Park, Charlotte's first official green space, about 11 miles southeast of Charlotte's city center. Along this trail and in the vicinity you encounter tennis courts, horseshoe pits, picnic shelters, five expansive soccer fields, a pond stocked for fishing, and the city's first leash-free dog park, Ray's Fetching Meadows. Make sure to prepare if you wish to partake in any of these activities. The trail briefly follows an elevated board-walk that connects to the McAlpine Creek Greenway and runs past a pleasant pond and several soccer fields. The trail becomes wide and gravel and utilizes a section of the 5k cross-country course before veering off into the shade and returning to the pond and trailhead via the nature trail.

Route Details

Park your vehicle in McAlpine Creek Park's lot. Before you leave to hit the trail, consider that most of this trail is open to the sun and prone to insects and heat. Bring some sunscreen, bug spray, and plenty of liquids with you if you plan to spend a considerable amount of time on the trail or in the soccer fields. Walk to the trailhead, marked by a kiosk on the south side of the parking lot. A paved trail approximately 4 feet wide leads past a soccer field on your left and connects to an elevated concrete bridge that crosses a small stream. At the foot of the bridge is the intersection with the McAlpine Creek Greenway. Here, turn left (north) onto the paved greenway path toward the cross-country start line. Cross another concrete bridge over a small stream. Here the trail becomes gravel; to the left is a shaded area with benches and picnic tables, a very nice open-air auditorium, horseshoe pits, and barbecue grills. To the right is a pond stocked for fishing. The trail splits three ways. To the left a wooden footbridge returns to the parking lot, and to the right the trail follows the shore of the pond and heads to Ray's Fetching Meadows, where you can let your dog run around without the leash for a while.

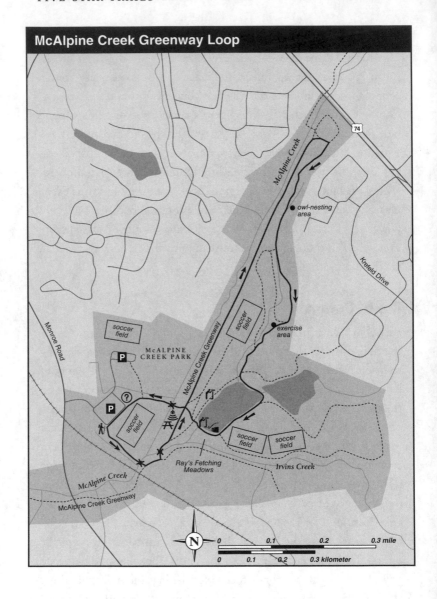

McAlpine Creek Greenway Loop

Here, the trail to the right that leads to Fetching Meadows is also the beginning of the 5k cross-country course, marked by blue and white mileage markers. Stay straight on the wide gravel greenway. The trail really opens up to the sun along this section and becomes very wide. Be alert for other runners and bikers on this portion. During the summer, definitely keep your eyes and ears open for a person pushing a small ice-cream cart along the greenway, who, besides selling sweet frozen treats, also has a stock of cold water and sports drinks. His prices are reasonable, too, so there's no reason for you to get dehydrated on this route. The greenway stretches far off in the distance here, the green grass of the surrounding fields and forest vividly contrasting with the light-tan 4-foot-wide gravel path. The trail is easy to follow, and you'll discover plenty of shady spots in the grass and under trees on the sides of the trail for a rest. Or sit on the sidelines of one of the park's five soccer fields, which are usually buzzing with local soccer matches or practice.

After 0.6 mile from the four-way junction, veer to the right (east) and follow the narrower 3-foot-wide gravel trail. The trail follows this bearing for approximately 40 feet and then turns right

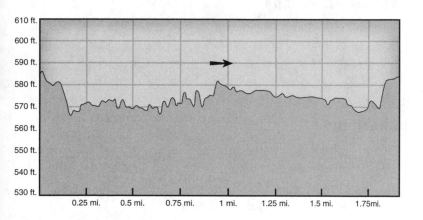

(south) in the direction of the fishing pond. This section of the trail is very shady and much cooler in temperature. The trail here also passes through an interesting owl-nesting site. This is a great birding area, so keep your eyes peeled and bring your binoculars to get a closer glimpse.

Walk for 0.4 mile until you reach an exercise area with pull-up bars, sit-up benches, and stretch bars on your right. Here the path splits in three directions again. Stay straight toward the pond. After 0.1 mile, stay right (east) along the shore of the pond. Benches are scattered along the pond shore and make a great spot to sit and watch the wading birds. Ahead on your left there are an observation deck and several picnic pavilions. From the observation deck you may see some of the local fish—including bass, crappie, catfish, and bream—that the anglers on the shore's edge are eager to reel in. It's fine to feed the fish here, but several signs warn against feeding the water-fowl. Several willow trees line the pond. Follow the trail around the pond and back to the elevated boardwalk. This boardwalk leads to the parking lot and the end of the trail at the kiosk.

Nearby Attractions

This greenway is largely surrounded by urban development. Around this area you find the usual suspects in fast-food and big-box stores at the nearby Quorum Marketplace and the Independence Square East Shopping Center.

Directions

From the Charlotte city center, take US 74 East toward NC 24 and follow it for 5.4 miles. Turn right onto Idlewild Road and follow it for 0.2 mile. Turn left onto Monroe Road. Follow Monroe Road for 2.6 miles to McAlpine Creek Park, on the left.

McAlpine Creek Park: Pond Loop

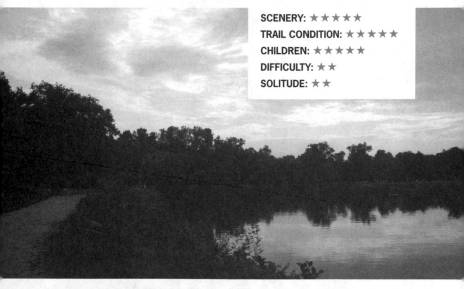

SCENERY: ★ ★ ★ ★ ★
TRAIL CONDITION: ★ ★ ★ ★ ★
CHILDREN: ★ ★ ★ ★ ★
DIFFICULTY: ★ ★
SOLITUDE: ★ ★

A PONDSIDE I VIEW N McALPINE CREEK PARK

GPS TRAILHEAD COORDINATES: N35° 9.051' W80° 44.609'

DISTANCE & CONFIGURATION: 1.4-mile balloon

HIKING TIME: 2 hours

HIGHLIGHTS: Pond, fishing pier, observation deck, dog park, horseshoes, picnic pavilion, and soccer fields

ELEVATION: 583' at the trailhead to 569' at lowest point

ACCESS: Daily, sunrise–sunset

MAPS: At Charlotte Visitor Info Center, trailhead kiosk, and **parkandrec.com**

FACILITIES: Restrooms and water fountains

WHEELCHAIR ACCESS: Yes, on paved paths around pond and to restrooms

COMMENTS: Dogs are allowed; the trail is shared with runners, walkers, and bikers.

CONTACTS: (704) 432-1570; **parkandrec.com**

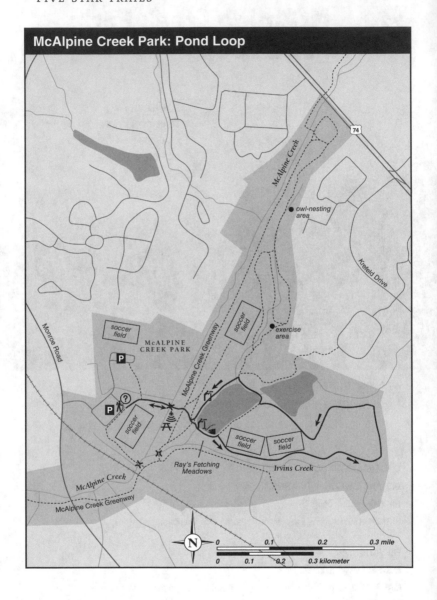

McAlpine Creek Park: Pond Loop

Overview

This shorter route through McAlpine Creek Park follows a section of the greenway and loops around a nice pond. The trail runs in very close proximity to Ray's Fetching Meadows, a leash-free dog park, and is a great trail for kids. The elevation is almost nonexistent except for climbing a few stairs to get on and off the elevated boardwalk, and the distance is short enough to keep their attention and not wear out the youngest of children. The loop is very much out in the open, and the park is often moderately busy, providing an element of safety. The pond is open for fishing from the shore or the railed observation deck. An abundance of waterfowl wading and splashing in the pond provides an extra element of wonder for kids and adults alike.

Route Details

Park your vehicle in McAlpine Creek Park's lot and walk to the kiosk and trailhead in the northeast corner of the parking lot. Follow the gravel 6-foot-wide path along the back side of the soccer field that leads to the elevated wooden boardwalk. The boardwalk crosses a small stream and leads to the larger gravel McAlpine Creek Greenway. Be alert for bikers and runners with whom you'll be sharing this popular greenway, especially if you have small children. At the foot of the boardwalk are a picnic area on the right with tables, an open-air amphitheater, horseshoe pits, barbecue grills, and benches beside the stream. Just straight ahead and to the right is a spacious dog park called Ray's Fetching Meadows, the first leash-free dog park in all of Charlotte, and it is very popular with those who live in this area south of Charlotte's city center. A good number of benches dot the dog park, so you have plenty of places to rest while your mutt runs circles around you. If you did bring children, make sure to keep your ears open for the snack vendor who walks up and down the greenway selling water, sports drinks, and, most importantly, sweet ice-cream treats. Just listen for the bells.

Stay straight (southeast) and cross the small arching foot-bridge near the edge of the pond shore. Follow the path along the pond's edge. After 350 feet from the start of the pond shore, you reach a split in the trail. To the left the path continues along the lake shore. Turn right and follow the sign toward the South Fields. This section of the trail skirts the edge of several soccer fields. Follow the trail along the southern soccer field. You'll likely find an energetic and exciting game or practice going on, and there are plenty of shady spots in the grass under the trees at the field's edge where you can sit and watch. Usually families and friends will be grouped together with coolers and sometimes barbecue grills doing a bit of tailgating in support of their favorite young soccer players. If the fields are open, they're a great place to throw a baseball, football, or Frisbee, or even have a soccer match of your own. Just past the soccer fields, to the left, several small birdhouses sit back off the trail in the shady forest. This is a good spot for bird-watching, and the interpretive plaques throughout this forested and shaded section describe the variety of

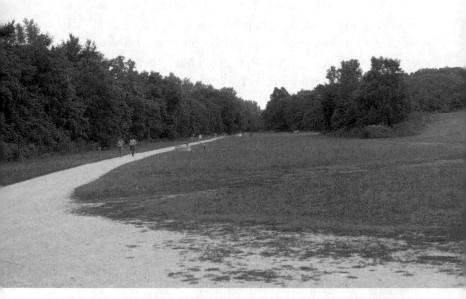

THE WIDE-OPEN FIELDS ALONG THE TRAIL GET PLENTY OF RECREATIONAL USE.

bird species you're likely to encounter. For better viewing, bring a pair of binoculars for you and the kids, if you brought them along. Follow the trail and it will curve back toward the pond. The trail passes the soccer fields again, this time on the left, before running alongside a large wetland area on the right. More interpretive plaques highlight the different birdlife that you are likely to see in the wetlands compared with that you'd see in the forest. Follow the trail through the wetland and back to the pond.

After 0.7 mile from the trail junction at the edge of the pond shore, you reach the shore again and are likely to find people fishing on the pond's edge, as well as a good number of waterfowl wading in the pond and looking for an easy meal from hikers. Several signs here advise that it's fine to feed the fish but ask that you not feed the waterfowl. Turn right (north) to circle back around the pond shore, passing the observation deck on your left. To your right is the elevated boardwalk that you can cross again to return to the trailhead and kiosk.

Nearby Attractions

This greenway is largely surrounded by urban development. Around this area you find the usual suspects in fast-food and big-box stores at the nearby Quorum Marketplace and the Independence Square East Shopping Center.

Directions

From the Charlotte city center, take US Highway 74 East toward NC 24 and follow it for 5.4 miles. Turn right onto Idlewild Road and follow it for 0.2 mile. Turn left onto Monroe Road. Follow Monroe Road for 2.6 miles to McAlpine Creek Park, on the left.

23 McDowell Nature Preserve: Trail Combo 1

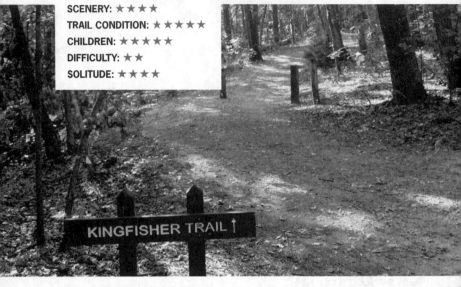

SCENERY: ★ ★ ★ ★
TRAIL CONDITION: ★ ★ ★ ★ ★
CHILDREN: ★ ★ ★ ★ ★
DIFFICULTY: ★ ★
SOLITUDE: ★ ★ ★ ★

THE KINGFISHER TRAIL LEADS THE WAY TO LAKE WYLIE AT McDOWELL NATURE PRESER'

GPS TRAILHEAD COORDINATES: N35° 5.909' W81° 1.530'

DISTANCE & CONFIGURATION: 2.5-mile loop

HIKING TIME: 2 hours

HIGHLIGHTS: Lake Wylie, fishing pier, primitive campsites, and Diane Schumpert Memorial Garden

ELEVATION: 667' at the trailhead to 709' to 562' at lowest point

ACCESS: Daily, 7 a.m.–sunset; campsites are $12–$22

MAPS: At the park visitor center, trailhead kiosks, or **parkandrec.com**

FACILITIES: Restrooms, water fountains, bathhouse, and kayak rentals

WHEELCHAIR ACCESS: This hike is not wheelchair-accessible; the Four Seasons Trail is the only accessible trail in the park.

COMMENTS: The campground office closes at 4:30 p.m. Monday–Friday. If you're interested in camping here or hiking into the primitive campsites, get to the park before the office closes. The campground and access to the trail are gated and locked at sunset.

CONTACTS: (704) 583-1284; **parkandrec.com**

Overview

Take a walk through one of the most popular sections of McDowell Nature Preserve on a loop hike that connects three different trails in the park. The hike leads through a slightly hilly hardwood forest and follows along the shore of Lake Wylie before entering back into the forest and climbing over some moderate hills in the park. Along this trail you will also find several primitive campsites for visitors who prefer a secluded wilderness experience. The backpacking sites are available for reservation online or from the campground office.

Route Details

This trail begins at the parking lot that serves the primitive campsites located at the back of the campground. Enter the park and follow the sign to the campground. The campground is well marked, and signs will direct you to the trailhead and the large primitive-campground parking lot. The Kingfisher Trailhead is in the northwest corner of the lot, where a brown wooden sign identifies the 4-foot-wide gravel trail. The trail is blazed with white and black signs with an image of a hiker on them. Follow the trail into the hardwood forest, and after 50 feet you pass the first of seven primitive campsites along this section of the hike. The primitive sites are exceptionally close to the trailhead, so the hike really isn't too bad if you have decided to backpack your gear into the sites. This trail combination is a good introduction to wilderness camping and backpacking for those who are just getting started. The best part is that if you forget something, your car is never far away. Each primitive site has tent pads, picnic tables, and fire rings.

After passing the last primitive campsite, continue on the trail, passing a small wooden fence and continuing slightly downhill. After 0.1 mile from the start of the trail, you reach a spur trail on your left (west) leading down to Lake Wylie and a fishing pier there. This is a nice side trip. Stay straight (north) where the trail becomes a narrower dirt path and you begin to catch glimpses of the lake through

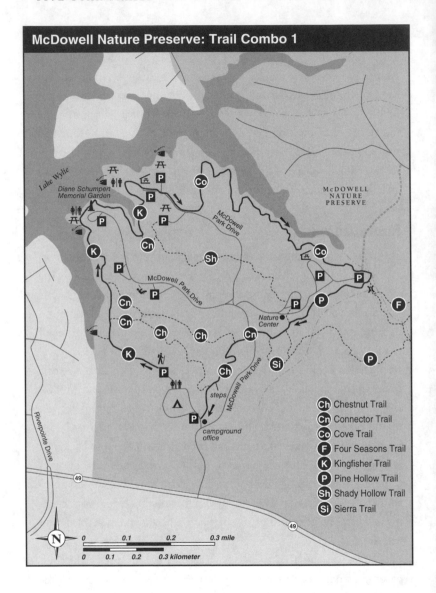

McDowell Nature Preserve: Trail Combo 1

Lake Wylie

Diane Schumpert Memorial Garden

McDowell Park Drive

McDowell Park Drive

McDowell NATURE PRESERVE

Nature Center

McDowell Park Drive

Riverpointe Drive

steps

campground office

49

49

Ch Chestnut Trail
Cn Connector Trail
Co Cove Trail
F Four Seasons Trail
K Kingfisher Trail
P Pine Hollow Trail
Sh Shady Hollow Trail
Si Sierra Trail

N

0   0.1   0.2   0.3 mile

0   0.1   0.2   0.3 kilometer

the trees. After just 250 feet from the junction with the spur trail that leads to the pier, you come to the junction with a spur leading to Chestnut Trail. Stay on the Kingfisher Trail straight (north). The trail begins to follow along the lakeshore, and along this section beautiful large houses line the opposite shore. Here several small sand beaches along the lakeshore make for excellent swimming, sunning, and picnic areas. Continue on the trail, passing a large boathouse on the left. Continue for 0.1 mile from the junction with the spur trail that leads to the Chestnut Trail until you reach a gravel road. Follow this gravel road uphill for 450 feet until you reach a set of steps on the left that lead into the forest on a narrower dirt path. Here the Kingfisher Trail is much smaller and feels much more natural than the previous section.

After 0.1 mile the Kingfisher Trail leads to a sandy point with a pavilion, a large observation deck, and a floating pier. Restrooms, kayak rentals, picnic tables, and water fountains make this a great spot to spend the afternoon exploring the lake. Pass the observation deck on the left and continue on the concrete path along the lakeshore lined with lampposts, which keep the path lit nicely at night.

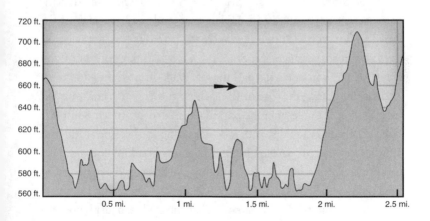

The area becomes more landscaped as you pass through the Diane Schumpert Memorial Garden, where several benches offer excellent lake views. After passing the covered swing on your right, head uphill to rejoin the Kingfisher Trail, which continues along the lakeshore and becomes a dirt path again. After 50 feet you pass a sandy beach on your left, and along this section the trail skirts the shore of one of the lake's arms, which is lined with more long stretches of sandy beaches. After 0.1 mile from the pavilion and observation deck, the trail turns left (north), continuing on Kingfisher Trail uphill and along the lakeshore.

The hillside you encounter at this point of the trail is a little tricky. Multiple trails have been carved along this section, most of them leading to the same place or down to the lake and back to the real trail. The abundance of paths makes the real trail hard to find and follow. Keep your eye out for trail markers, and look for improvements such as branches that block spur trails in an effort to curb this problem and the hillside erosion that it creates. After the trail clearly becomes a single path, wooden steps lead downhill to a small wooden footbridge before the trail climbs back uphill and passes a picnic area on the left. Continue through the forest until you reach the large covered picnic pavilion. After 0.1 mile from the left turn and the beginning of the uphill section, you will reach a gravel road. Turn right (east) and follow the gravel road, passing restrooms and water fountains on your right. After 300 feet you arrive at a parking lot. Walk through the parking lot and continue along the road until reaching the Cove Trail on your left (north) after 0.1 mile from the parking lot. Turn left (north) onto the Cove Trail. Follow the dirt path 0.7 mile along the lakeshore and past another large picnic pavilion before reaching a parking lot and road. Cross the parking lot and begin hiking on the paved Four Seasons Trail. Follow the paved Four Seasons Trail for 50 feet and then turn right (west) onto the Pine Hollow Trail at the trailhead just before the paved bridge with wooden handrails.

The Pine Hollow Trail heads uphill and follows alongside the main park road until you reach the nature center. After 0.2 mile from the point where you joined the Pine Hollow Trail, turn left (west), passing a fire ring surrounded by benches. After 300 feet you reach a junction with a white-blazed connector trail. Go straight (west) onto the connector trail and cross a paved road. After 500 feet from the beginning of the connector trail, you will reach a junction with the Chestnut Trail. Turn left (south) onto the Chestnut Trail, which leads down a steep hill. Continue on the Chestnut Trail for 0.1 mile until you reach a set of wooden steps on the left. Follow the wooden steps to the left that lead to the campground office, parking lot, trailhead, and the end of the hike 500 feet away. From here you can follow the road to the right to return to the primitive-camping parking lot where you began your hike or follow the road back to your campsite.

Nearby Attractions

Charlotte's city center is only 20 minutes to the north. The nature preserve has a campground and a nature center that is definitely worth exploring. The campsites include water, electricity, a picnic table, and a tent pad and are suitable for tents or RVs; primitive sites are also available. McAlpine Creek Park (see pages 140 and 145) offers more hiking 23 miles to the east toward Charlotte. To the north, 15 minutes or 10 miles away, is Daniel Stowe Botanical Garden (see page 174).

Directions

From the Charlotte city center, take I-277 South/US 74 West and follow it for 0.8 mile. Merge onto I-77 South/US 21 South via Exit 1B toward Columbia and follow it for 3.4 miles. Take the NC 49 South exit, Exit 6B, toward Airport/South Tryon Street and follow it for 0.3 mile. Turn right onto South Tryon Street/NC 49. Continue to follow NC 49 south for 10.3 miles until you reach McDowell Nature Preserve, on the right.

McDowell Nature Preserve: Trail Combo 2

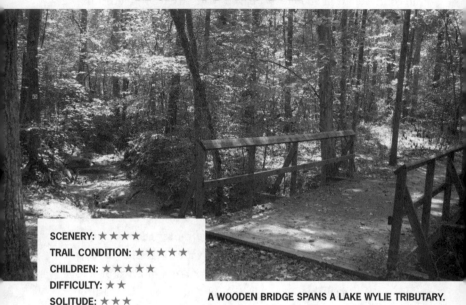

SCENERY: ★ ★ ★ ★
TRAIL CONDITION: ★ ★ ★ ★ ★
CHILDREN: ★ ★ ★ ★ ★
DIFFICULTY: ★ ★
SOLITUDE: ★ ★ ★

A WOODEN BRIDGE SPANS A LAKE WYLIE TRIBUTARY.

GPS TRAILHEAD COORDINATES: N35° 6.031' W81° 1.201'

DISTANCE & CONFIGURATION: 2.2-mile loop

HIKING TIME: 1.5 hours

HIGHLIGHTS: McDowell Nature Preserve Nature Center, creek-side hiking, and challenging hills

ELEVATION: 678' at the trailhead to 592' at lowest point

ACCESS: Daily, 7 a.m.–sunset

MAPS: At the park's nature center, trailhead kiosks, or **parkandrec.com**

FACILITIES: Restrooms, water fountains, bathhouse, and kayak rentals

WHEELCHAIR ACCESS: This hike is not wheelchair-accessible; the Four Seasons Trail is the only accessible trail in the park.

COMMENTS: The campground office closes at 4:30 p.m. Monday–Friday. If you're interested in camping here or hiking into the primitive campsites, get to the park before the office closes. The campground and access to the trail are gated and locked at sunset.

CONTACTS: (704) 583-1284; **parkandrec.com**

Overview

After checking out the preserve's nature center, access this loop hike—a great trail for birding—that connects three popular trails. Preserve volunteers have established an abundance of bird boxes to help promote avian life in the surrounding forest. After exploring the hardwood forest around the nature center, the trail follows alongside a small creek with a rocky streambed, reminiscent of streams in the farther west Appalachian Mountains. The short path is a nice warm-up trail in the morning. It starts out with a gradual climb and then, after reaching the stream and following level ground, encounters several challenging hills that really get the blood pumping before you return to the nature center.

Route Details

Walk to the kiosk in front of the nature center—this marks the beginning of the trail. A connector trail runs beside the nature center and past several benches, compost bins, a water tank, and picnic tables before reaching the Pine Hollow Trail junction after 200 feet. Turn right (west) and follow the Pine Hollow Trail for 80 feet around the nature center, passing a fire ring surrounded by several benches until you reach a trail junction. Keep left (southwest) heading toward the Sierra Trail Loop. After 50 feet, the start of the trail is well marked with a sign. Follow the Sierra Trail Loop downhill until you reach the Pine Hollow Trail at the bottom of the hill and turn left (east).

The trail continues downhill and runs beside a small stream that is concealed for the most part within a deep gully. There are many bird boxes or birdhouses along this section of the trail. Birders should keep binoculars close at hand on this section of the trail. The path crosses a small footbridge spanning a stream before ascending a small hill and passing several benches. The trail is nicely constructed with simple wooden steps in the exceptionally steep areas of this section. The pleasant hike traverses up and down small hills through a dense and shaded forest.

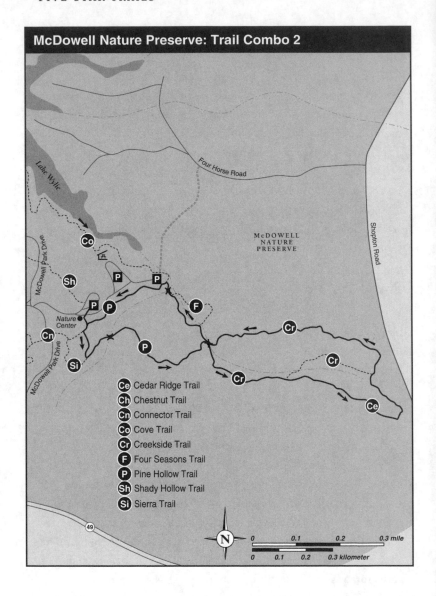

McDowell Nature Preserve: Trail Combo 2

Ce Cedar Ridge Trail
Ch Chestnut Trail
Cn Connector Trail
Co Cove Trail
Cr Creekside Trail
F Four Seasons Trail
P Pine Hollow Trail
Sh Shady Hollow Trail
Si Sierra Trail

After 0.03 mile from where you joined the Pine Hollow Trail, you reach a wide wooden bridge that crosses a beautiful stream with a rocky creek bed. Turn right (east) onto the Creekside Trail after crossing the bridge. The trail does what the name implies, following alongside the creek, which is a perfect place to turn over rocks and search for salamanders. After another 120 feet you reach a junction for the Creekside Trail. Stay to the right (south) and cross the wooden bridge spanning a creek tributary. After following alongside the creek, the trail passes under power lines and through the clearing they create before returning back into the forest.

Continue along the Creekside Trail for 0.2 mile from the point where you originally joined the trail until you reach the Cedar Ridge Trail. Continue straight (east) to join the Cedar Ridge Trail, which climbs up a considerable hill before leveling out on a ridge and then gradually descending to rejoin the Creekside Trail after 0.5 mile. Turn right (north) onto the Creekside Trail, which passes through a section of dense cedar trees with fairly level ground; it's a nice break from the hills behind you. Continue for 0.5 mile on the Creekside Trail until you reach the Pine Hollow Trail again at the wooden bridge you crossed

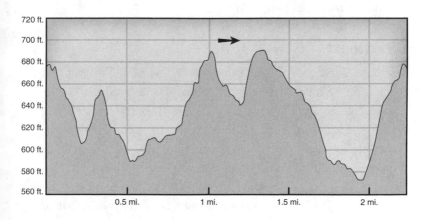

earlier. Turn right (north) and follow the Pine Hollow Trail for 130 feet until you reach the paved Four Seasons Trail. Turn left (west) and follow the paved path along the creek. After 0.1 mile, the Four Seasons Trail splits in two directions. Stay to the left (northwest) and continue for another 230 feet, passing the small clearing with picnic tables that sit to your left alongside the stream. Cross the concrete bridge with wooden rails and turn left (west) onto the Pine Hollow Trail, following it uphill for 0.2 mile until you reach the nature center again. Once behind the nature center, take the spur trail to the right that you came in on, which leads alongside the nature center and returns to the parking lot, the trailhead, and the end of the trail.

Nearby Attractions

Charlotte's city center is only 20 minutes to the north. The nature preserve has a campground and a nature center that is definitely worth exploring. The campsites include water, electricity, a picnic table, and a tent pad and are suitable for tents or RVs. McAlpine Creek Park (see pages 140 and 145) offers more hiking 23 miles to the east toward Charlotte. To the north, 15 minutes or 10 miles away, is Daniel Stowe Botanical Garden (see page 174).

Directions

From the Charlotte city center, take I-277 South/US 74 West and follow it for 0.8 mile. Merge onto I-77 South/US 21 South via Exit 1B toward Columbia and follow it for 3.4 miles. Take the NC 49 South exit, Exit 6B, toward Airport/South Tryon Street and follow it for 0.3 mile. Turn right onto South Tryon Street/NC 49. Continue to follow NC 49 south for 10.3 miles until you reach McDowell Nature Preserve, on the right. Drive into the park and follow the signs to the nature center. You'll see an entrance station, but drive past it. Park in the lot just past the nature center.

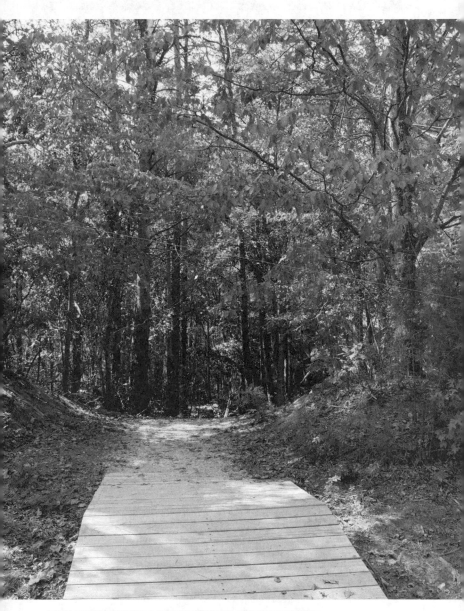

A WALKWAY CROSSES A BOGGY SECTION OF THE PRESERVE.

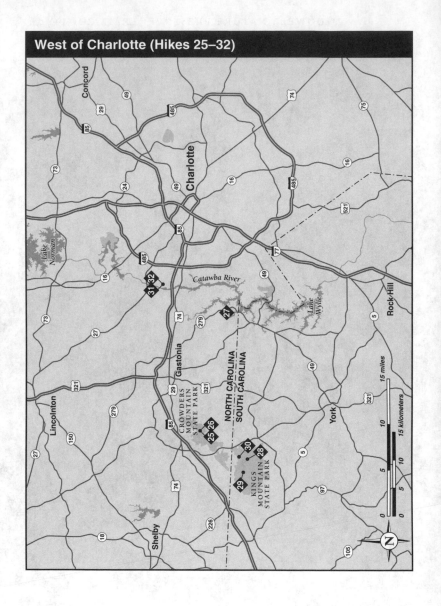

West of Charlotte (Hikes 25–32)

West of Charlotte

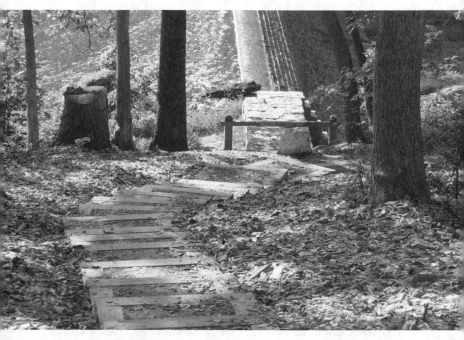

A STEEP TRAIL LEADS DOWN TO THE CRAWFORD LAKE DAM, ALONG THE
HISTORIC FARM TRAIL AT KINGS MOUNTAIN STATE PARK.

25

Crowders Mountain State Park: Lake Loop

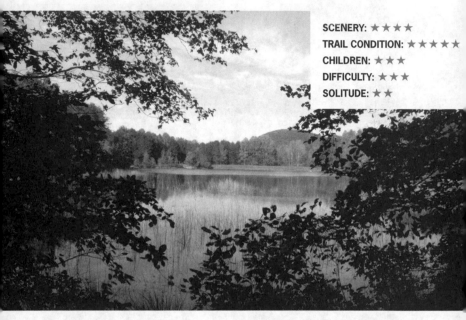

SCENERY: ★ ★ ★ ★
TRAIL CONDITION: ★ ★ ★ ★ ★
CHILDREN: ★ ★ ★
DIFFICULTY: ★ ★ ★
SOLITUDE: ★ ★

A BEAUTIFUL VIEW OF AN UNNAMED LAKE IN CROWDERS MOUNTAIN STATE PARK

GPS TRAILHEAD COORDINATES: N35° 12.824' W81° 17.605'

DISTANCE & CONFIGURATION: 3.3-mile loop

HIKING TIME: 2 hours

HIGHLIGHTS: Lake, family campground, rock formations, and creek

ELEVATION: 889' at the trailhead to 1,100'

ACCESS: Daily, 8 a.m.–6 p.m.; campsite $13 per night; acquire camping permit at visitor center

MAPS: At visitor center, trailhead kiosk, and **ncparks.gov**

FACILITIES: Restrooms, walk-in campsites, water fountains and spigots, picnic shelters, and amphitheater

WHEELCHAIR ACCESS: None of the trails have it, although the visitor center is wheelchair-accessible.

COMMENTS: This is a very popular park; to avoid crowds, consider hiking on weekdays and avoiding holidays. The trails in the park are popular for running, so be aware of runners and give them the right-of-way.

CONTACTS: (704) 853-5375; **ncparks.gov**

Overview

This hike combines the Pinnacle, Turnback, Fern, and Lake trails to create a loop that traverses a wide variety of landscapes. The highlight is at the end of the trail, when the Fern and Lake trails loop around a picturesque lake and cross several creeks. At the beginning of the route, the trail ascends more than 200 feet in the first mile, climbs to a ridge, and then steeply descends to the lake. The route is not nearly as challenging as the hike up to the summit of Crowders Mountain. If you want to turn your quick and pleasant day hike into an overnight camping trip under the stars, the Pinnacle Trail leads to a spur trail that heads to the walk-in camping sites.

Route Details

A kiosk to the left of the visitor center, or the northeast corner of the lot, marks the trailhead of a spur trail, a 4-foot-wide dirt path through a beautiful forest, that leads to the Crowders and Pinnacle trails. After 0.1 mile, the trail splits. Turn left (west) onto the orange circle–blazed Pinnacle Trail heading toward the family campground.

Continue for 0.5 mile until you reach a split in the trail. To the right (north), the trail leads to the family campground. The large campground has 10 well-spaced primitive sites, each equipped with a picnic table and a tent pad, with a nice buffer for sound and privacy. A small privy has the charm of an old-fashioned outhouse with water spigots. The best part about the backcountry campground is that the dry, prechopped firewood is free. Stay to the left (southwest) and continue on the Pinnacle Trail, blazed with orange circles. The trail gradually ascends to an area of the trail that traverses through a rocky section lined with boulders and interesting rock formations.

After 0.4 mile turn left (east) onto the Turnback Trail. The trail leaves the large boulders and the ridge behind and descends steeply toward the lake. After 0.7 mile of traveling downhill, you'll begin to see a parking lot through the trees, and 20 yards later you'll reach the junction with the Fern Trail. Turn right (south) onto the 2-foot-wide

Crowders Mountain State Park: Lake Loop

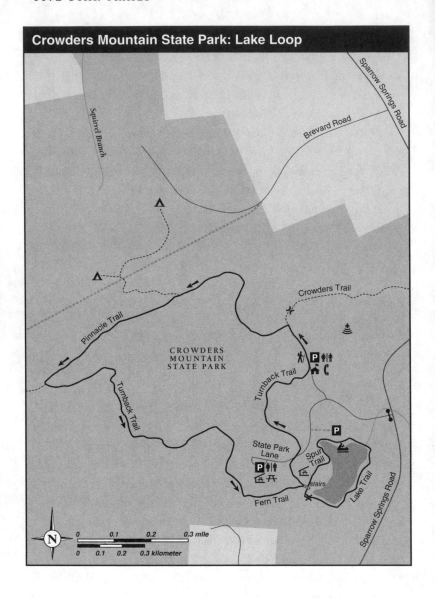

Fern Trail, blazed with red hexagonal signs, and follow it 0.3 mile. On this section, the trail descends to a stream that winds through the forest. The path follows alongside the creek and climbs a small hill to the intersection with the Lake Trail. The Fern Trail ascends a small wooden staircase to the left, but you'll stay straight (southeast) on the Lake Trail, continuing on the path that follows alongside the creek and crosses the wooden footbridge, to the left.

After crossing the bridge, the Lake Trail turns immediately to the left (east) and follows the opposite side of the stream. You quickly reach a picturesque lake, and the trail loops around the lakeshore. Plenty of benches and small clearings line this pretty section of trail.

Continue around the lake for 0.7 mile from the junction where you continued straight on the Lake Trail until you reach a spur trail leading to the picnic area. Turn right (northwest) onto this spur, which leads uphill, climbing a series of simple wooden steps. After walking 150 feet and reaching the top of the hill, turn left (west) onto the wider path. The path descends to the Fern Trail–Lake Trail junction after 350 feet. Turn right (northwest) and continue on the Fern Trail toward the park's main road, State Park Lane, following the trail uphill on the wooden steps for 450 feet. At the top of the hill, the trail

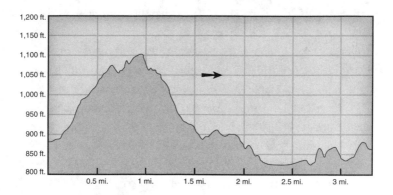

exits into a parking lot. Walk across the parking lot toward the stop sign. Turn right (northeast) and walk to the trail, crossing 380 feet down the road. Cross the paved road here and continue on the Fern Trail. After 0.1 mile you reach the Turnback Trail. Turn right (north) and continue for 0.3 mile through the forest until you reach the trailhead, parking lot, and the end of the trail.

Nearby Attractions

Just 17 miles to the southwest, Kings Mountain State Park (see pages 184 and 189) offers horseback riding and hiking trails; the terrain at Kings Mountain is much easier to traverse than that at Crowders Mountain. The paved trail at adjoining Kings Mountain National Military Park (see page 179) features monuments to the Battle of Kings Mountain, where American forces won their first major battle against the British in the Revolutionary War. Also nearby and just 20 miles to the east is the Daniel Stowe Botanical Garden (see page 174).

Directions

From I-85 South, take Exit 13 to Edgewood Road. At the top of the ramp, turn left onto Edgewood Road. At the first stoplight, turn right onto Franklin Boulevard/US 74 and drive about 2 miles. At the next stoplight, turn left onto Sparrow Springs Road. Continue on Sparrow Springs Road for approximately 2 miles, and turn right again on Sparrow Springs Road. The main entrance to the park will be on the right in less than 1 mile. Park your vehicle in the visitor-center lot.

From I-85 North, take Exit 8 to NC 161. At the top of the ramp, turn right onto NC 161 and drive about 0.25 mile. Then turn left onto Lake Montonia Road/Pinnacle Road and follow it to its end at Sparrow Springs Road. Turn left at the stop sign onto Sparrow Springs Road. The main entrance to the park will be on the left in about 1 mile. Park your vehicle in the visitor-center lot.

26

Crowders Mountain State Park: Trail Combo

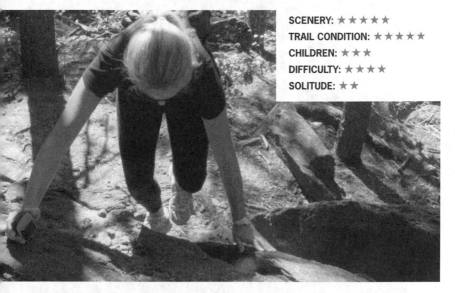

SCENERY: ★ ★ ★ ★ ★
TRAIL CONDITION: ★ ★ ★ ★ ★
CHILDREN: ★ ★ ★
DIFFICULTY: ★ ★ ★ ★
SOLITUDE: ★ ★

A HIKER SCRAMBLES UP A STEEP BUT SHORT SECTION OF ROCK ALONG THE TRAIL.

GPS TRAILHEAD COORDINATES: N35° 12.832' W81° 17.620'

DISTANCE & CONFIGURATION: 5-mile balloon

HIKING TIME: 3 hours

HIGHLIGHTS: Crowders Mountain overlook, rock formations, and challenging trail

ELEVATION: 929' at the trailhead to 1,552'

ACCESS: Daily, 8 a.m.–6 p.m.

MAPS: At visitor center, trailhead kiosk, and **ncparks.gov**

FACILITIES: Restrooms, walk-in campsites, water fountains and spigots, picnic shelters, and amphitheater

WHEELCHAIR ACCESS: None of the trails have it, although the visitor center is wheelchair-accessible.

COMMENTS: This is a very popular park; to avoid crowds, consider hiking on weekdays and avoiding holidays. The trails in the park are popular for running, so be aware of runners and give them the right-of-way.

CONTACTS: (704) 853-5375; **ncparks.gov**

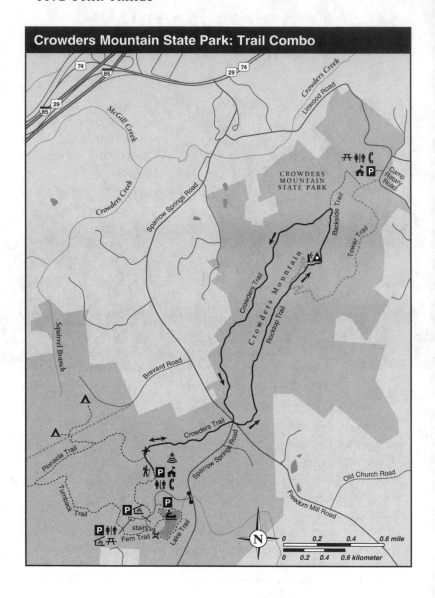

Crowders Mountain State Park: Trail Combo

Overview

This hike combines three trails in Crowders Mountain State Park—the Crowders Trail, Rocktop Trail, and Backside Trail—to create a loop that climbs challenging hills up to the summit of Crowders Mountain. Although the summit isn't all that impressive because it's covered with communication towers, the surrounding rock formations, outcrops, and views of the surrounding mountains are worth the hike. It's definitely not easy or short at more than 4 miles, so consider your fitness level and allow plenty of time to hike the trail based on how fit you are. The best views on the hike are when the forest opens up or a rock formation juts out to the east and gives you a view of the Charlotte skyline rising out of the forest in the distance.

Route Details

A kiosk to the left of the visitor center, or the northeast corner of the lot, marks the trailhead of a spur trail that leads to the Crowders Trail. Walk straight (north) on the spur trail for 0.2 mile until the trail splits. To the left (west) is the Pinnacle Trail. Stay right (northeast)

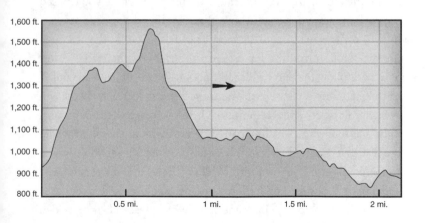

on the Crowders Trail. The trails in the park are very well maintained, and the Crowders Trail is well blazed with white diamonds. The trail descends through a beautiful hardwood forest to a small wooden footbridge that crosses a narrow creek. The path curves to the right and then intersects with the park's main paved road after 0.5 mile. It's slightly confusing here, as the trail also splits at this paved road intersection. The Crowders Trail is straight ahead and the Rocktop Trail is to the right (southeast) about 60 feet. Cross the road and continue on the Rocktop Trail, blazed with red circles.

From the Rocktop Trailhead the trail begins to climb upward immediately, and as you climb the trail becomes more and more rocky. As the trail ascends, you find yourself climbing short but very steep sections of rock. There are plenty of easy ways to get up and over these small boulders and rock sections, something most people can handle. At the top of the first hill, you reach a rocky outcrop with views of the surrounding mountains. The best view is to the right (east), where you can see the skyline of Charlotte in the distance rising out of the forest. It's really an amazing perspective of the city.

The trail descends from the outcrop and crosses a gravel road—the blue-blazed Tower Trail, 1.0 mile from where you crossed the park's main paved road. Cross the gravel road and stay straight (north) on the red-blazed Rocktop Trail for 0.2 mile that ascends the rocky hill in front of you. Stay to the right of the gravel Tower Trail and follow the orange-blazed Backside Trail, which leads uphill to three soaring radio, television, and cell-phone towers that sit on the summit of Crowders Mountain. Once you reach the towers, turn right and follow the concrete path around them, at the point where the dirt trail descends toward the lookout. After 90 feet you come to an incredible stone outcrop with excellent views to the west and east and a better view of the Charlotte skyline. Explore the lookout area before continuing on the Backside Trail, which descends the wooden stairs behind the lookout.

After 0.3 mile, turn left (southwest) onto the white-blazed Crowders Trail, descending into the forest. From here, it's an easy and well-marked hike that gradually descends and crosses the main road after 1.7 miles. Continue straight on the Crowders Trail for 0.8 mile to the parking lot, the trailhead, and the end of the trail.

Nearby Attractions

Just 17 miles to the southwest, Kings Mountain State Park (see pages 184 and 189) offers horseback riding and hiking trails; the terrain at Kings Mountain is much easier to traverse than that at Crowders Mountain. The paved trail at adjoining Kings Mountain National Military Park (see page 179) features monuments to the Battle of Kings Mountain, where American forces won their first major battle against the British in the Revolutionary War. Also nearby and just 20 miles to the east is the Daniel Stowe Botanical Garden (see page 174). A highlight of the garden is the conservatory that houses an impressive collection of orchids and other tropical plants.

Directions

From I-85 South, take Exit 13 to Edgewood Road. At the top of the ramp, turn left onto Edgewood Road. At the first stoplight, turn right onto Franklin Boulevard/US 74 and drive about 2 miles. At the next stoplight, turn left onto Sparrow Springs Road. Continue on Sparrow Springs Road for approximately 2 miles, and turn right again on Sparrow Springs Road. The main entrance to the park will be on the right in less than 1 mile. Park your vehicle in the visitor-center lot.

From I-85 North, take Exit 8 to NC 161. At the top of the ramp, turn right onto NC 161 and drive about 0.25 mile. Then turn left onto Lake Montonia Road/Pinnacle Road and follow it to its end at Sparrow Springs Road. Turn left at the stop sign onto Sparrow Springs Road. The main entrance to the park will be on the left in about 1 mile. Park your vehicle in the visitor-center lot.

27

Daniel Stowe
Botanical Garden

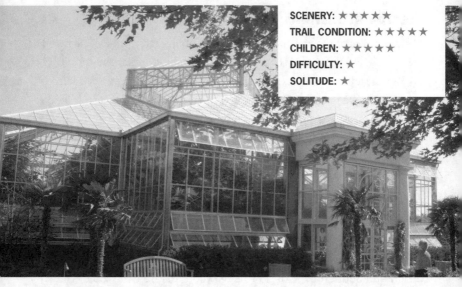

SCENERY: ★ ★ ★ ★ ★
TRAIL CONDITION: ★ ★ ★ ★ ★
CHILDREN: ★ ★ ★ ★ ★
DIFFICULTY: ★
SOLITUDE: ★

THE IMPRESSIVE ORCHID CONSERVATORY AT DANIEL STOWE BOTANICAL GARDEN

GPS TRAILHEAD COORDINATES: N35° 10.066 W81° 3.468

DISTANCE & CONFIGURATION: 0.6-mile loop

HIKING TIME: 2 hours

HIGHLIGHTS: Conservatory, orchid display, fountains, sculptures, and gardens

ELEVATION: Negligible—653' at the trailhead to 644' at the lowest point

ACCESS: Daily, 9 a.m.–5 p.m.; adults $12, seniors age 60 or older $11, children ages
4–12 $11, free for members and children under age 4

MAPS: At the garden visitor center and **dsbg.org**

FACILITIES: Restrooms, museum, and water fountains

WHEELCHAIR ACCESS: Yes.

COMMENTS: Plan to spend considerable time at the gardens—more than you would
on a normal hike of this length. There's so much to see packed in such a
small space. The gardens are very popular, so to avoid crowds, explore on
weekdays and avoid holidays.

CONTACTS: (704) 825-4490; **dsbg.org**

Overview

If you love gardens, plan on spending the whole day for this walk. The route explores the best features of the gardens, including the Formal Display Gardens and the four Perennial Gardens. Daniel Stowe, a textile CEO, set aside 400 acres of his estate and funded Charlotte's best botanical gardens, which fully opened to the public on October 9, 1999. This route stops in at the highlight of the garden: the Orchid Conservatory, the only glass-house conservatory in the Carolinas open to the public, which debuted on January 19, 2008. The garden is filled with traditional and modern architecture and sculpture, as well as a collection of beautifully constructed fountains that are certain to capture the imagination; walk under the arching fountain at the risk of getting very wet. The garden is well suited for both kids and adults, and the trails and grounds are immaculately maintained by what are considered to be among the finest gardeners in the region.

Route Details

The visitor center offers maps with your entrance purchase, and the route starts from the redbrick path that runs behind the impressive stained glass domed visitor center. Turn left (southeast) and follow the redbrick path, passing under the East Pergola and heading straight (southeast) for the conservatory 200 feet away. A path leads to the left inside the conservatory and passes by a wonderful collection of orchids housed in glass boxes. Around the corner you pass an impressive wall with water cascading down the front and orchids clinging to it, protected by small alcoves of rock. It's an amazing display, masterfully constructed and designed.

A pebble path leads through the conservatory, where you can explore an entire collection of tropical plants, and then exits the conservatory. Once you've left the conservatory, stay straight (northwest), heading to the East Pergola again, and once under the arbor, turn left (southwest). Walk for 40 yards under the arbor, and once you reach the hedge-lined brick path, turn right (northwest). Continue

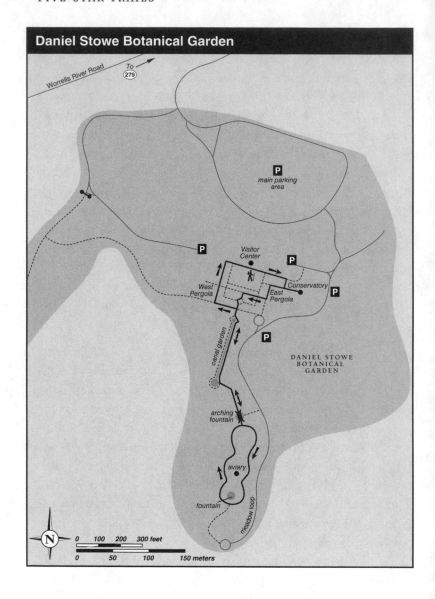

for 90 feet and reach the diamond-shaped fountain in the Cottage Garden. Turn left (east) and follow the path down a set of stairs, continuing straight (southwest) and following the path alongside the Canal Garden. Continue along the long path that follows alongside the channel of water and arrive at the large circular fountain after 500 feet. Turn left (southeast) on the brick paved walkway and follow the path through the Allée Garden. The trail passes under a spectacular fountain that arches over the walkway and turns on without warning. It also turns off without any warning at all. If you're walking on the path or you happen to be under the fountain when the fountain decides to turn off—say, when you're getting a picture of the waters arching over your head—you're going to get soaked. This is great in the heat of a Charlotte summer if you're dressed accordingly and not wielding any expensive electronics, not so much in winter or when you're carrying a thousand-dollar camera. Signs warn you about the fountain, but keep your eyes open because it's easy to get distracted by the beautiful flowers and trees around the fountain and walk right in to an unexpected soaking. Two large wooden chairs nearby are perfect for a rest; take time to watch children and spectators playing in the fountain waters.

After you pass the fountain, stay to the left (east), passing under arching bushes and walking past a small aviary with a variety of birds housed inside. The junction with the meadow loop arrives in just 120 feet. The meadow loop is to the left (south) and travels for 0.5 mile through the meadow in the north section of the garden. Stay straight (west), following the path around the fountain and back toward the aviary. Continue back to the arching fountain and continue the way you came in along the water channel. Once you reach the end of the water channel at 320 feet from the last fountain, turn left (northwest) and follow the paved path about 60 feet to the West Pergola. Turn right (northeast) and head toward the visitor center, walking under the West Pergola. After 60 feet, you reach the redbrick path that runs directly in front of the visitor center. Turn right (southeast) to walk to the visitor center and the end of the route.

Nearby Attractions

Downtown Charlotte, the historic Fourth Ward district, and many of the city's greenway trails are 20 miles to the east of the gardens. The closest town for restaurants and provisions is Belmont, North Carolina, 6 miles to the north of the gardens. More hiking trails and other adventurous outdoor activities can be found at the U.S. National Whitewater Center (see pages 194 and 199), 14 miles to the north of the gardens. The center has more than 20 miles of hiking and biking trails, a man-made river with rapids used to train professional whitewater rafters from around the world (open to the public), kayaking, zip-line courses, rope courses, and a climbing wall. Get the best of both worlds and have a civilized and cultured morning at the gardens and then head to the center for an afternoon of rollicking adventure and high adrenaline activity.

Directions

Daniel Stowe Botanical Garden is 21 miles west of Charlotte at the North Carolina–South Carolina state line, outside the town of Belmont, North Carolina. From the Charlotte city center, take I-277 South for 0.9 mile. Merge onto Freedom Drive via Exit 1A toward US 29/NC 27 and follow it for 2.5 miles. Merge onto I-85 South via the ramp on the left toward Gastonia and follow it for 7.7 miles. Take the NC 273 Exit 27, toward Belmont/Mt. Holly and follow it for 0.3 mile. Turn left onto NC 273/Park Street/Beatty Drive and continue to follow NC 273 for 2 miles. Turn left onto South Central Avenue/NC 273 and continue to follow NC 273 for 4.1 miles. Turn right onto Armstrong Road/NC 273 and follow it for 2.4 miles. Turn right onto South New Hope Road/NC 279 and follow for 0.7 mile. Daniel Stowe Botanical Garden will be on your left. After driving down a winding road that passes a pond, park in the main lot.

28

Kings Mountain National Military Park: Battlefield Trail

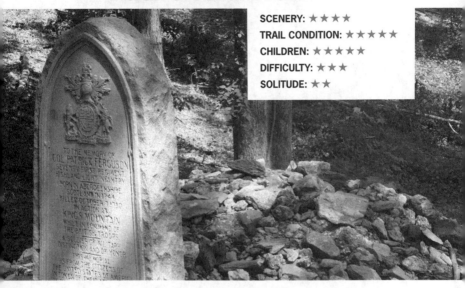

SCENERY: ★ ★ ★ ★
TRAIL CONDITION: ★ ★ ★ ★ ★
CHILDREN: ★ ★ ★ ★ ★
DIFFICULTY: ★ ★ ★
SOLITUDE: ★ ★

THIS STONE MEMORIAL FOR MAJOR PATRICK FERGUSON IS ONE OF MANY MONUMENTS COMMEMORATING THE HEROIC BATTLE THAT WAS FOUGHT AT KINGS MOUNTAIN NATIONAL MILITARY PARK.

GPS TRAILHEAD COORDINATES: N35° 8.483 W81° 22.557

DISTANCE & CONFIGURATION: 1.5-mile loop

HIKING TIME: 1.5 hours

HIGHLIGHTS: Battlefield monuments, interpretive plaques, and visitor center

ELEVATION: 852' at the trailhead to 1,002'

ACCESS: Monday–Friday, 9 a.m.–5 p.m.; Saturday–Sunday, 9 a.m.–6 p.m.

MAPS: At the park's visitor center, trailhead kiosks, and **nps.gov/kimo**

FACILITIES: Visitor center, restrooms, water fountains, and campground

WHEELCHAIR ACCESS: Yes, though steep in places; use caution.

COMMENTS: This trail can have high use on weekends in the summer. Avoid crowds by hiking during other times.

CONTACTS: (864) 936-7921; **nps.gov/kimo**

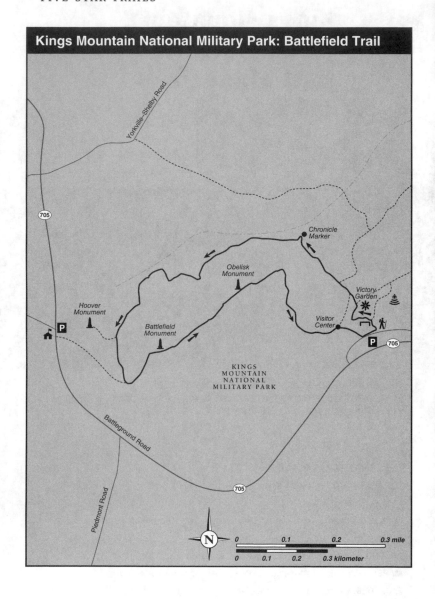

Kings Mountain National Military Park: Battlefield Trail

Overview

Explore the site of what is considered one of the most important conflicts of the Revolutionary War. This paved, wheelchair-accessible trail explores the 1780 Battle of Kings Mountain through a very well-done collection of interpretive plaques and monuments. The beautiful hardwood-forest setting and occasional distant views along the trail, which circles the top of Kings Mountain, are worth the trip even if you're not interested in the history. One of the highlights is an obelisk, reminiscent of the Washington Monument, that marks the location in which the Battle of Kings Mountain began to turn in favor of the revolutionary patriots.

Route Details

Watch the 26-minute video at the visitor center to get an overview of the historical significance of the battlefield through which the trail goes. The Battlefield Trail starts from the trailhead on the north side of the parking lot, 100 yards to the right (east) of the visitor center. The entire trail is paved and wheelchair-accessible. Benches to the left

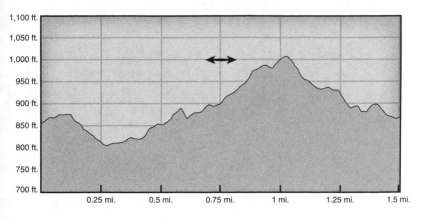

(west) of the trail overlook a clearing and the visitor center. Continue on the trail past the amphitheater on the right (east), and after 30 yards the trail splits. Stay to the left toward the visitor center. After 50 feet you reach another junction. To the left is the visitor center. Turn right (east) away from the visitor center and onto the Battlefield Trail, passing the Victory Garden on the right. The trail begins to circle the base of Kings Mountain and enters a thin hardwood forest. After an additional 50 feet, a spur trail leads to the left (west). Stay straight (north) and continue on Battlefield Trail. Here you'll find the first of many interpretive plaques (complemented by a free cell-phone audio tour) that explore the progression of the battle. A phone number, printed on each of the kiosks, connects you to a recording that explains the feature or location you are currently exploring.

Stay straight on the main paved path and pass a replica of the gravestone that marks the burial site of Major William Chronicle, Captain John Mattocks, William Rabb, John Boyd, and Major Patrick Ferguson. The original gravestone, weathered and barely readable, sits next to the replica. The paved path runs beside a stream, crossing over it several times. All the bridges crossing the stream are concrete and wheelchair-accessible. The trail winds through the forest, and benches at regular intervals offer resting spots. After 0.7 mile a spur trail leads to the right (east) to the Hoover Monument marking the 150th anniversary of the battle at Kings Mountain, where in 1930 President Herbert Hoover gave a speech commemorating the event. Take a side trip and then return to the main trail, continuing straight on the main path. As the trail circles around to the left (west), it climbs steeply uphill; at the top of the hill, you're rewarded with views of distant ridges through the trees. The trail continues to climb a second hill, and after 0.2 mile from the Hoover Monument spur trail, you reach the Battlefield Monument, a four-sided column that commemorates the battle in the words of Thomas Jefferson: "Here the tide of the battle turned in favor of the American Colonists." At this point, it's easy to imagine every rock on the hillside surrounding the trail as marking the grave of a soldier and every scar on the trees in the forest as being a mark made from the bullets of British and patriot men who fought in this battle.

The trail leads downhill for 0.2 mile to another monument—an obelisk closely resembling the Washington Monument, yet much smaller. This towering obelisk commemorates the victory of the Kings Mountain battle and lists the American forces that participated in the battle. From here the trail continues downhill for another 50 feet to a stone column that marks the exact spot where Major Ferguson, the British commander, fell on October 7, 1780. The trail then climbs steeply uphill to the visitor center, marking the end of the trail.

Nearby Attractions

Kings Mountain State Park (see next two profiles) adjoins Kings Mountain National Military Park. Many more miles of hiking trails, as well as a campground, are located in the state park. Cowpens National Battlefield is just outside of Gaffney, South Carolina, 30 miles west of Kings Mountain National Military Park. About an hour to the west, near Hendersonville, North Carolina, you can visit the home of poet, writer, and editor Carl Sandburg.

Directions

From Greenville, South Carolina, travel on I-85 North to NC Exit 2. Merge onto Banks Road, and then take the first right onto Battleground Road/NC 216. Follow Battleground Road for 3.2 miles to the park visitor center.

From Charlotte, travel on I-85 South to NC Exit 2. Turn left onto Battleground Road/NC 216 and travel for 3.2 miles to the park visitor center.

29 Kings Mountain State Park: Historic Farm Trail

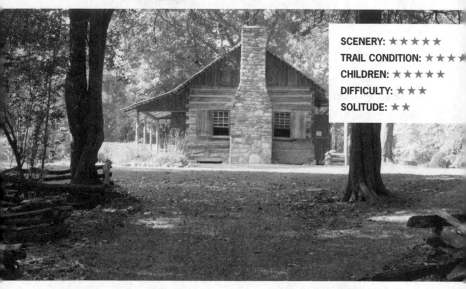

SCENERY: ★ ★ ★ ★ ★
TRAIL CONDITION: ★ ★ ★ ★
CHILDREN: ★ ★ ★ ★ ★
DIFFICULTY: ★ ★ ★
SOLITUDE: ★ ★

THIS LOG CABIN IS AMONG THE ATTRACTIONS AT KINGS MOUNTAIN'S LIVING HISTORY FARM.

GPS TRAILHEAD COORDINATES: N35° 8.937' W81° 20.725'

DISTANCE & CONFIGURATION: 1.6-mile out-and-back

HIKING TIME: 2 hours

HIGHLIGHTS: Lake Crawford, Civilian Conservation Corps building, and Living History Farm

ELEVATION: 752' at the trailhead to 841'

ACCESS: Daily, 8 a.m.–6 p.m.; Daily, 7 a.m.–9 p.m. during daylight saving time; adults $2, South Carolina senior citizens $1.25, free for children age 15 and younger

MAPS: At the park visitor center for $1, trailhead kiosks, and **southcarolinaparks.com**

FACILITIES: Restrooms and water fountains

WHEELCHAIR ACCESS: None

COMMENTS: The Living History Farm can be busy on summer weekends, so to avoid crowds, hike the trail at other times. The trail from Lake Crawford to the Living History Farm is fairly well maintained; when trees are down, they are mostly cleared, and most people will be able to get around or over them.

CONTACTS: (803) 222-3209; **southcarolinaparks.com**

Overview

Walk along the shore of Lake Crawford and through a hardwood forest to a very interesting Living History Farm. The Living History Farm re-creates of what life was like in the 1800s, around the time that the battle on Kings Mountain was fought. There are gardens, chicken coops, blacksmith stations, and cabins to explore. It's a self-guided tour most of the year. If your imagination is easily captured and you have even an inkling of an interest in history, be prepared to spend more time than you would expect wandering around this excellent farm museum. A large conference center, artfully constructed of stone and built by the Civilian Conservation Corps during the Great Depression, also sits along the shore of Lake Crawford.

Route Details

The Historic Farm Trailhead is on the south side of the parking lot, just to the right (southwest) of the conference center. Take the 6-foot-wide, wood chip–covered trail downhill toward the lake. A series of staircases makes traversing the steep hill easy. Walk past the lake dam and a picnic table. From the perspective on the trail, it appears that the trail crosses the dam, but it actually doesn't. The trail veers to the right (south), continues along the back side of the dam, and reaches a creek behind the dam. Large boulders and rocks make easy crossing of the creek.

The trail becomes somewhat confusing here. Stay parallel with the dam and look for the yellow blazes on the trees that lead you up the hill straight ahead (southeast). The trail curves to the east and continues running parallel to the shore of Lake Crawford. Forty yards ahead, the trail splits. To the left, the trail stays along the shore of the lake. Stay right and follow the trail into the forest and away from the lake. The Historic Farm Trail is much better maintained than most of the other trails in the state park, mostly because of this trail's popularity. When trees are downed, they are cleared, unlike many of the other trails where you have to climb over downed

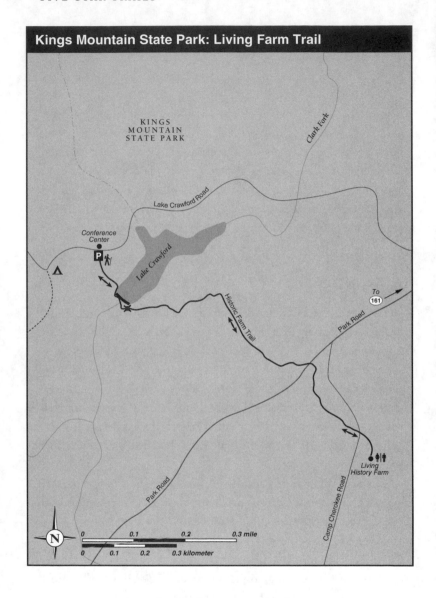

Kings Mountain State Park: Living Farm Trail

trees. Continue on the trail, crossing over a small tributary stream via a wooden footbridge. The trail begins to level out, and the path becomes wider and easier to follow in this section, where you also encounter a lot of exposed granite. Continue along the path until you reach the park's main paved road, after 0.5 mile from the beginning of the trail. The trail continues on the other side. It's easily visible and marked by a rustic fence. Continue through the pine grove and under power lines. After 0.2 mile stay straight (southeast), and cross the road that leads to the gravel parking lot for the Living History Farm. A small rustic cabin on your right has restrooms inside. Walk just past the cabin and turn right (south) down the gravel path lined with a rustic wooden fence leading to the Living History Farm. The gravel trail ends at a kiosk, where you will find a map and additional information, in front of the Living History Farm exhibit. From here you can explore the loom, chicken coop, cabin, blacksmith shop, cotton mill, sorghum manufacturing station, woodcraft shop, and garden of herbs, collards, and corn. Don't forget that the animals, including horses, donkeys, and goats, are all the way to the left (southeast) side of the farm. When you are finished exploring the farm, just turn

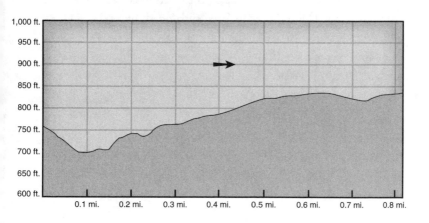

around and walk back the way you came in, along the yellow-blazed Historic Farm Trail, which will take you back to Lake Crawford, the trailhead, and the parking lot.

Nearby Attractions

The state park offers miles of hiking trails (see next profile), and the campground offers RV and tent sites, as well as small rustic cabins for rent. Kings Mountain National Military Park (see previous profile), just a few miles north, also has several trails worth exploring. The national park has a very nice visitor center with an informative movie on the rich history of the area shown every half-hour.

Directions

From I-85, take Exit 8, and turn left onto NC 161. Cross the North Carolina–South Carolina state line; the park entrance will be on the right. Drive toward Lake Crawford Campground, on the north side of the park's main paved road. Follow the signs to the Historic Farm Trailhead and park in the large parking lot.

From I-77, take Exit 77 for SC 5 toward Rock Hill. Follow SC 5 through Rock Hill to York. In York, turn north onto US 321, and then bear left onto SC 161. The park entrance will be on the left. Drive toward the Lake Crawford Campground on the north side of the park's main paved road. Follow the signs to the Historic Farm Trailhead and park in the large parking lot.

Kings Mountain State Park: Trail Combo

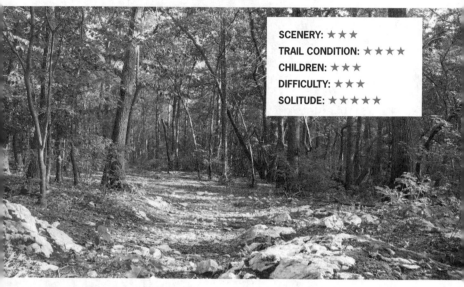

SCENERY: ★ ★ ★	
TRAIL CONDITION: ★ ★ ★ ★	
CHILDREN: ★ ★ ★	
DIFFICULTY: ★ ★ ★	
SOLITUDE: ★ ★ ★ ★ ★	

YOU'LL FIND INTERESTING MOUNDS OF EXPOSED ROCK ALONG THE RIDGELINE TRAIL.

GPS TRAILHEAD COORDINATES: N35° 8.127' W81° 21.029'

DISTANCE & CONFIGURATION: 5.4-mile balloon

HIKING TIME: 3.5 hours

HIGHLIGHTS: Creeks, boulders, mature forest, and solitude

ELEVATION: 792' at the trailhead to 850'

ACCESS: Daily, 8 a.m.–6 p.m.; Daily, 7 a.m.–9 p.m. during daylight saving time; adults $2, South Carolina resident seniors $1.25, free for children age 15 and younger

MAPS: At the park visitor center for $1, trailhead kiosks, and **southcarolinaparks.com**

FACILITIES: Restrooms

WHEELCHAIR ACCESS: None

COMMENTS: Be prepared with a map; there may not be other hikers along the trail to help you find your way if you get lost. The trail is also shared with horseback riders. In the event that you do encounter someone, he or she will probably be on horseback. Be respectful and give horses the right-of-way.

CONTACTS: (803) 222-3209; **southcarolinaparks.com**

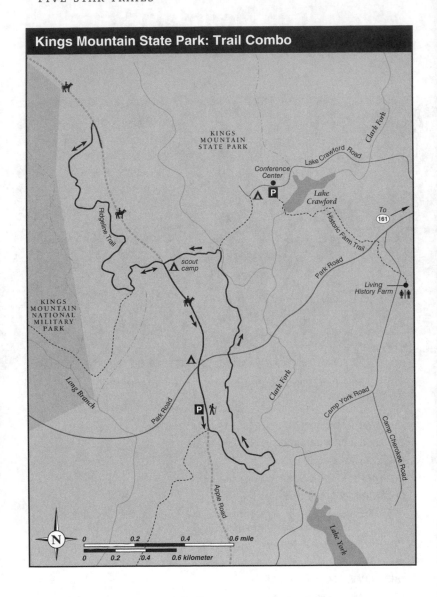

Kings Mountain State Park: Trail Combo

Overview

Exploring more than 5 miles of the backcountry of Kings Mountain State Park, this trail also ventures into nearby Kings Mountain National Military Park for a short distance. The trail is mostly a challenge in distance. It traverses a few demanding hills, but most of the path has hardly noticeable elevation. The trail offers a long and pleasant hike through a quiet and mature forest while crossing over several gentle streams and through two primitive group camps. *Note:* Stop at the visitor center to buy a decent trail map for $1. (The park offers free maps online and at the kiosks, but they're almost completely useless for hiking.)

Route Details

Walk to the gravel road and turn right (south). Walk about 50 feet until you reach the junction with the Hiking Trail, marked by a wooden post with a blue square, that crosses the main road, Apple Road. Turn left (east) onto the Hiking Trail.

The beginning section of the trail is not very well maintained, but the path is used often enough and well blazed, making it fairly

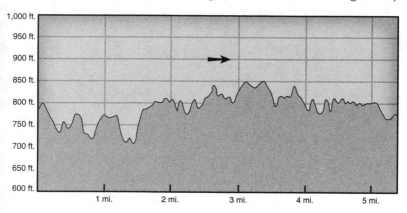

easy to follow. Just keep your eyes peeled for the painted blazes, and you'll make it through the few downed trees and very short overgrown sections. The first mile of the trail is fairly level until the trail gradually descends to a small creek. Along this section of the trail you will see plenty of exposed quartz, and around the creek bed you'll pass through large exposed boulders.

Hike for 0.8 mile until you cross the park's main paved road. Continue following the blue blazes through a quiet and mature forest, as the trail climbs over several hardly noticeable hills and runs alongside a slow-moving creek.

The trail crosses the creek via a small wooden footbridge and then continues through the forest, climbing over more pleasant rolling hills. After 0.5 mile, the trail splits. The trail to the right (northeast) leads to Lake Crawford and the campground there. Stay to the left and continue on the Hiking Trail toward Kings Mountain National Military Park. The trail climbs a steep hill through exceptionally dense forest, and after 0.3 mile you will reach a scout camp with picnic tables, water spigots, and fire rings. Directly after the scout camp, the trail crosses an old fire road. After 0.3 mile, a sign and a long wooden bench mark the junction with the Ridgeline Trail. Turn right (northwest) onto the Ridgeline Trail, marked with red square blazes. During this section the trail passes through interesting sections of exposed rock. Follow the Ridgeline Trail for 1.1 miles until you reach an unmarked junction with the old fire road.

Turn around and head back the way you came in on the Ridgeline Trail until you reach the junction with the Hiking Trail. Turn left (east) onto the Hiking Trail back to the scout camp and turn right (south) onto the old fire road toward the horse trailer parking lot. Along the gravel fire road, you pass through several large group camping sites with picnic tables, fire rings, and several simple restrooms. Stay straight on the gravel fire road for 0.4 mile until you reach the park's main paved road, Apple Road. Cross the paved road and continue on the gravel road on the other side of the street. Follow the gravel road back to the horse trailer parking lot and the trailhead where you started.

Nearby Attractions

The state park offers miles of hiking trails (see previous profile), and the campground offers campsites for RV and tent campers, as well as small rustic cabins for rental. Kings Mountain National Military Park (see page 179), just a few miles north, also has several trails worth exploring. The national park has a very nice visitor center with an informative movie on the rich history of the area shown every half-hour.

Directions

From I-85, take Exit 8, and turn left onto NC 161. Cross the North Carolina–South Carolina state line; the park entrance will be on the right. Park in the gravel horse-trailer lot on the south side of the main park road, between the road that leads to the Living History Farm and the border of Kings Mountain National Military Park.

From I-77, take Exit 77 for SC 5 toward Rock Hill. Follow SC 5 through Rock Hill to York. In York, turn north onto US 321, and then bear left onto SC 161. The park entrance will be on the left. Park in the gravel horse-trailer lot on the south side of the main park road, between the road that leads to the Living History Farm and the border of Kings Mountain National Military Park.

U.S. National Whitewater Center: Lake Loop

SCENERY: ★ ★ ★ ★
TRAIL CONDITION: ★ ★ ★ ★ ★
CHILDREN: ★ ★ ★ ★
DIFFICULTY: ★ ★
SOLITUDE: ★

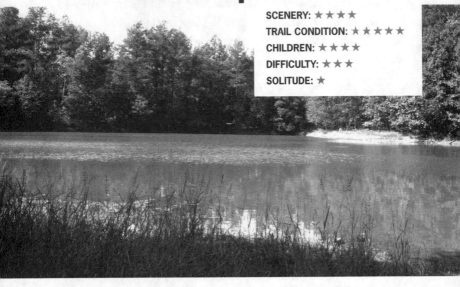

SEVERAL PONDS LIE ALONG THIS ROUTE AT THE U.S. WHITEWATER CENTER.

GPS TRAILHEAD COORDINATES: N35° 16.204' W81° 0.263'

DISTANCE & CONFIGURATION: 3.2-mile balloon

HIKING TIME: 2.5 hours

HIGHLIGHTS: Whitewater Center and lakes

ELEVATION: 657' at the trailhead to 693'

ACCESS: Daily, sunrise–sunset; $5 parking

MAPS: At the visitor center for $2

FACILITIES: Restrooms, water fountains, showers, whitewater rafting course, climbing wall, zip line, and ropes course

WHEELCHAIR ACCESS: The trails don't have it, but the Whitewater Center and many of the other facilities are accessible.

COMMENTS: The Whitewater Center is very popular, and the surrounding trails are often used by mountain bikers as well as hikers. The center allows you to bring water and trail snacks to accompany your hike (or bike ride), but no full picnics are allowed, as food and beverages are sold in the grill and gift shop. Avoid crowds by visiting the center during the week and by avoiding holidays.

CONTACTS: (704) 391-3900; **usnwc.org**

Overview

The trails that surround the whitewater course and the sprawling center traverse rolling hills bordered by the Catawba River and dotted with lakes. A steep hill near the beginning of the trail descends to level walking, and a steep hill toward the end of trail climbs back up to the trailhead.

Note: This route combines the South Trail and the Lake Loop in the southern section of the Whitewater Center to create a balloon hike that is also a favorite for mountain bikers. Stay alert, as some bikers like to push the speed barriers around the trails' hills and tight turns. Obviously, you should give a biker the right-of-way in most cases, as a matter of safety and common sense. To enhance visibility and reduce the chance of accidents, this route leads hikers in the opposite direction from that in which bikers will be riding.

Route Details

A green flag marks the trailhead, on the opposite side of the parking lot, at the Adventure Pavilion. It's easy to find even though the parking lot is huge, a testament to the popularity of this place.

Follow the 2-foot-wide gravel trail that runs under power lines and downhill for 0.1 mile to a split in the trail. To the right (northwest) is the blue square–blazed North Main Trail. Stay left (southwest) on the green circle–blazed Lake Loop Trail. After 300 feet, the trail splits again. Stay to the left (southeast) on the Lake Loop Trail. From here follow the trail for 0.1 mile until you reach another split in the trail. Stay to the left. The trail signs will direct you to stay to the right, but this is the direction in which the bikers are traveling, so it's safer for hikers to walk in the opposite direction to lower the risk of collisions. The trail from this point is extremely easy to follow and very well marked. The trail meanders through the forest for 0.8 mile, passing a large meadow on the left and crossing a gravel road before descending to the first of three lakes on the loop. The trail follows along the lakeshore and curves around two more lakes, zigzagging for 1.8 miles

U.S. National Whitewater Center: Lake Loop

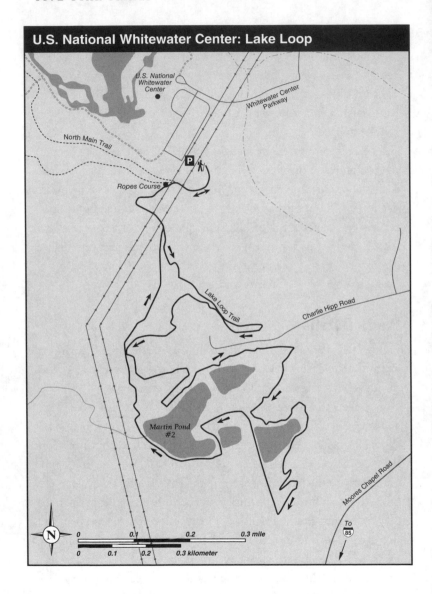

as it continues back toward the parking lot. Interestingly, each lake the trail passes varies in size and shape. The trail during this section even follows along a leveled berm that passes between two nearby lakes. After the trail leaves the lakes, it crosses under power lines and a clearing before rejoining the first junction, where the signs instruct which direction bikers should ride and where the Lake Loop Trail crosses the blue-blazed South Main Trail. Stay straight (northwest) on the Lake Loop Trail and continue toward the clearing in front of you. Continue for 0.1 mile until you reach the second junction with the South Main Trail. Turn right (northeast). Walk for 300 feet until you reach the junction with the North Main Trail. Turn right (east) and cross under the power lines. After 0.1 mile you reach the parking lot and trailhead at the top of the hill.

Nearby Attractions

The U.S. National Whitewater Center was built to train professional whitewater-rafting teams from around the world, but most of the time it hosts Charlotte locals, families, and outdoor adventurers looking for their next adrenaline fix. There are truly an astounding number of activities to explore in and around the center. It's home to the world's largest man-made whitewater river and also offers kayaking, mountain biking, rock climbing, zip lines, a canopy tour, and ropes courses.

The Daniel Stowe Botanical Garden (see page 174), 7 miles to the southeast of the Whitewater Center, is a great place to spend the day or just a couple of hours. The highlight of the garden is a conservatory with a large display of orchids and other exotic tropical plants. Downtown Charlotte, greenway hikes around the city, and the historic Fourth Ward (see page 32) are just 11 miles to the southeast of the Whitewater Center.

Directions

The U.S. National Whitewater Center is 11 miles (about 15 minutes) northwest of the Charlotte city center. From Downtown Charlotte, head west on US 74 West/Wilkinson Boulevard. Turn left onto I-485 Inner North Ramp and continue onto I-485 North/Statesville. Take Exit 12 for Moores Chapel Road and follow signs for USNWC. Once through the main gates, turn right toward the rear parking lot.

From Charlotte/Douglas International Airport, after exiting the airport, head west on US 74 West/Wilkinson Boulevard. Turn left onto I-485 Inner North Ramp and continue onto I-485 North/Statesville. Take Exit 12 for Moores Chapel Road and follow signs for USNWC. Once through the main gates, turn right toward the rear parking lot.

From I-85, head toward the intersection of I-485 and I-85 on the west side of Charlotte. Take Exit 29 for Sam Wilson Road and follow signs for USNWC. Once through the main gates, turn right toward the rear parking lot.

From I-485 head toward the intersection of I-485 and I-85 on the west side of Charlotte. Take Exit 12 for Moores Chapel Road and follow signs for USNWC. Once through the main gates, turn right toward the rear parking lot.

U.S. National Whitewater Center: North Main Trail

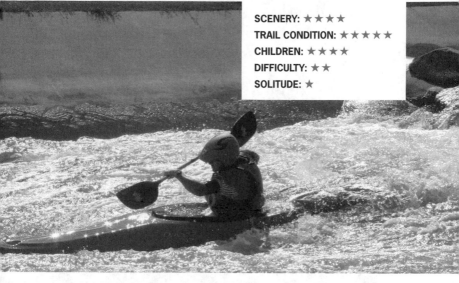

SCENERY: ★ ★ ★ ★
TRAIL CONDITION: ★ ★ ★ ★ ★
CHILDREN: ★ ★ ★ ★
DIFFICULTY: ★ ★
SOLITUDE: ★

IF YOU HIKE THE TRAILS AT THE RIGHT TIME, YOU CAN CATCH WHITEWATER RAFTERS AND KAYAKERS BATTLING THE RAPIDS.

GPS TRAILHEAD COORDINATES: N35° 16.167' W81° 0.328'

DISTANCE & CONFIGURATION: 2.8-mile balloon

HIKING TIME: 2 hours, but allow more time if you're interested in kayaking the Catawba River.

HIGHLIGHTS: Catawba River, whitewater course, ropes course, and zip line

ELEVATION: 632' at the trailhead to 662' to 573' at lowest point

ACCESS: Daily, sunrise–sunset; $5 parking

MAPS: At the visitor center for $2

FACILITIES: Restrooms, water fountains, showers, and climbing wall

WHEELCHAIR ACCESS: The trails don't have it, but the Whitewater Center and many of the other facilities are accessible.

COMMENTS: The Whitewater Center is very popular, and the surrounding trails are often used by mountain bikers as well as hikers. The center allows you to bring water and trail snacks to accompany your hike (or bike ride), but no full picnics are allowed, as food and beverages are sold in the grill and gift shop. Avoid crowds by visiting the center during the week and by avoiding holidays.

CONTACTS: (704) 391-3900; **usnwc.org**

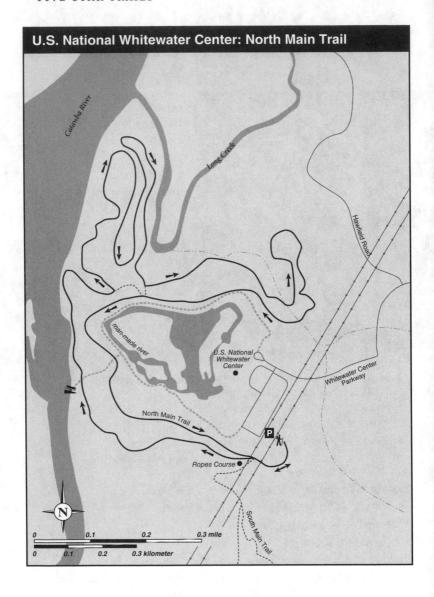

U.S. National Whitewater Center: North Main Trail

Overview

This popular route at the U.S. National Whitewater Center leaves from the main trailhead parking and follows the North Main Trail, exploring many of the outdoor-adventure opportunities you can experience while visiting the center. Along this path you'll pass under a fascinating ropes course, where you're likely to see adventurous folks working their way through the forest canopy, following the cables and ropes that guide them from platform to platform. From here the trail descends to the boat launch, where rafters and kayakers can access the Catawba River. The trail follows along the Catawba River and explores the surrounding forest before reaching the man-made river, where you can sit and watch whitewater rafters battle the rapids. Speeding over the whitewater river are those brave enough to tackle the high-speed zip line that stretches from the welcome center. You will follow along the man-made whitewater river before returning to the forest and then back to the trailhead where you started. The hike is easy and highly recommended. If you're the type to get bored with a hike through nothing but a forest, this is the trail for you. It will keep even the most easily bored among us captivated and interested in what comes around the next bend.

Route Details

The trailhead, marked by a green flag, is on the opposite side of the parking lot as the Adventure Pavilion. It's easy to find even though the parking lot is huge. From the parking lot, hike the spur trail to the junction with the North Main Trail and Lake Loop Trail. Stay to the right (east) on the North Main Trail. After 40 feet the trail splits. Stay left (northwest). Signs will direct bikers to the right, so hike the trail in the opposite direction to reduce the risk of collision with bikers.

After 30 feet you start to walk under the ropes course. There may be people walking above you, and this makes the trail especially interesting for children. The platforms built into the trees are obviously constructed by true craftsmen. Thirty feet after the ropes course, pass the junction with the South Main Trail and stay straight (west) on the North Main Trail. The trail descends to the U.S. National Whitewater Center flat-water launch, on the left. If you bought a pass from the visitor center to kayak on the Catawba, you can launch a kayak here.

Directly after the launch area, the trail crosses a gravel road and follows the Catawba River. This section of the trail is exceptionally nice. The trail ascends a small hill, and if the water is running you start to hear the rushing water of the rapids from the Whitewater Center. (The man-made river used to train whitewater rafters, as well as for recreation by all others, isn't always running.) The man-made river is on your right, to the east. Stay on the North Main Trail; do not take the exit trail marked on the map as an emergency access trail, unless you really want or need to cut the trail extremely short.

From here the trail descends to the Catawba River, where it's lined with ferns and other water-loving plants within the river corridor. A quarter-mile after reaching the river, a spur trail to the left leads down wooden steps to a short pier on the river. Stay straight and continue on the North Main Trail to the junction with the figure eight. The intersection is very easy to miss. Here, don't stay straight and don't cross the wood-plank footbridge—instead, curve to the right toward the signpost.

You quickly exit the forest and head under a NATIONAL WHITE-WATER CENTER sign, then exit onto the shore of the man-made river. Sit on the edge of the river and watch paddlers, rafters, and kayakers battle the rapids while people race down the zip line above to the platform straight ahead. Turn right (west) onto the gravel road and follow along the shore of the river for 400 feet, where the trail splits. Stay to the right (southwest) on the 1-foot-wide gravel trail that splits off from the larger main gravel road. Stay on the North Main Trail, which continues running along the shore of the man-made river. After 0.2 mile, turn right (south) and follow the North Main Trail uphill along the stone-covered path and back into the forest. From here the trail is easy to follow. Just stay on the North Main Trail for 0.5 mile, keeping straight at the junction with the North Main Trail, until you reach the trailhead, the parking lot, and the end of the trail.

Nearby Attractions

Activities abound at the Whitewater Center. The Daniel Stowe Botanical Garden (see page 174), 7 miles to the southeast of the Whitewater Center, is a great place to spend the day or just a couple of hours. The highlight of the garden is a conservatory with a large display of orchids and other exotic tropical plants. Downtown Charlotte, greenway hikes around the city, and the historical Fourth Ward (see page 32) are just 11 miles to the southeast of the Whitewater Center.

Directions

The U.S. National Whitewater Center is 11 miles (about 15 minutes) northwest of the Charlotte city center. From Downtown Charlotte, head west on US 74 West/Wilkinson Boulevard. Turn left onto I-485 Inner North Ramp and continue onto I-485 North/Statesville. Take Exit 12 for Moores Chapel Road and follow signs for USNWC. Once through the main gates, turn right toward the rear parking lot.

From Charlotte/Douglas International Airport, after exiting the airport, head west on US 74 West/Wilkinson Boulevard. Turn left onto I-485 Inner North Ramp and continue onto I-485 North/ Statesville. Take Exit 12 for Moores Chapel Road and follow signs for USNWC. Once through the main gates, turn right toward the rear parking lot.

From I-85, head toward the intersection of I-485 and I-85 on the west side of Charlotte. Take Exit 29 for Sam Wilson Road and follow signs for USNWC. Once through the main gates, turn right toward the rear parking lot.

From I-485 head toward the intersection of I-485 and I-85 on the west side of Charlotte. Take Exit 12 for Moores Chapel Road and follow signs for USNWC. Once through the main gates, turn right toward the rear parking lot.

Appendixes & Index

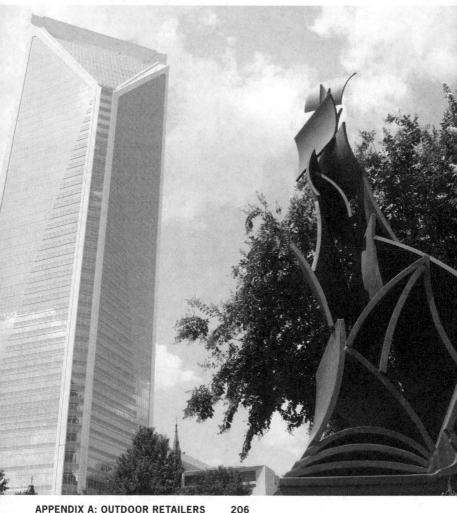

Appendix A: Outdoor Retailers

BASS PRO SHOPS
basspro.com
8181 Concord Mills Boulevard
Concord, NC 28027
(704) 979-2200

DICK'S SPORTING GOODS
dickssportinggoods.com
4325 Barclay Downs Drive
Charlotte, NC 28209
(704) 972-9400

GREAT OUTDOOR PROVISION CO.
greatoutdoorprovision.com
4341 Park Road
Charlotte, NC 28209
(704) 523-1089

JESSE BROWN'S ADVENTURE
jessebrowns.com
14825 Ballantyne Village Way, Suite 140
Charlotte, NC 28277
(704) 369-5140

JESSE BROWN'S OUTDOORS
jessebrowns.com
4732 Sharon Road
Charlotte, NC 28210
(704) 556-0020

OLD TOWN OUTFITTERS
153 East White Street
Rock Hill, SC 29730
(803) 324-9133

REI CHARLOTTE
rei.com
9755 Northlake Centre Parkway
Charlotte, NC 28216
(704) 921-0320

**U.S. NATIONAL WHITEWATER
CENTER OUTFITTER'S STORE**
usnwc.org
820 Hawfield Road
Charlotte, NC 28214
(704) 391-3900, ext. 203

Appendix B: Hiking Clubs

Many outdoor adventurers call the Charlotte area home. Consider these contacts for connecting with fellow hiking enthusiasts.

CAROLINA BERG WANDERERS
carolinabergs.com

CAROLINA MOUNTAIN CLUB
carolinamtnclub.org

CHARLOTTE HIKING MEETUP
meetup.com/hiking-charlotte

CHARLOTTE LADY HIKERS
meetup.com/charlotte-lady-hikers

CHARLOTTE OUTDOOR CLUB SOUTH
charlotte.outdoorclubsouth.com

Index

About the Author

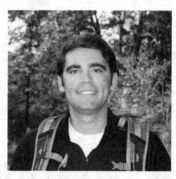

Joshua Kinser is a writer and musician based in Chimney Rock, North Carolina, about 45 minutes from Charlotte. He grew up on the beaches of Pensacola, Florida, but almost every summer he headed to the mountains of North Carolina to indulge his passions for hiking and backpacking. Desire for new experiences has led him to some of the coolest jobs in the world, which include writing hiking guidebooks.

Joshua has worked as a backcountry-wildlife biology field technician for the U.S. Forest Service on research projects studying amphibian populations, having joined teams in Hawaii's Volcanoes National Park, Montana's Glacier National Park, and the national-forest lands surrounding California's Yosemite National Park. He is a also a professional drummer who has performed in wedding bands, original acts, and international cruise-ship orchestras. Australia, China, Japan, Indonesia, New Zealand, and South Korea count among his stops.

Joshua is the author of Moon Travel Guides' *Florida Gulf Coast,* third edition. His articles have also appeared on websites such as Trails .com, eHow.com, and USA Today Travel, and in the *Pensacola News Journal.* He holds a degree in journalism from Pensacola State College.

Check out this other great title from
— Menasha Ridge Press! —

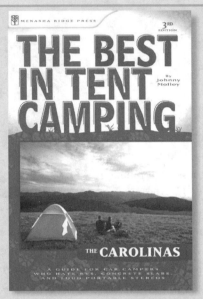

The Best in Tent Camping:
The Carolinas

by Johnny Molloy
ISBN: 978-0-89732-798-5
$15.95, 3rd edition

192 pages, 6x9, paperback
maps, photographs, index

In North Carolina, experience the rare spruce–fir forest of Balsam Mountain Campground or the sand dunes of Frisco Campground. Visit Cherry Hill, South Carolina's finest upcountry campground, or pitch your tent by the Atlantic Ocean in Hunting Island State Park. From the Smokies to the Atlantic, each campground profiled is unique. Perfect for those quick weekend trips, this guide packs well for easy access by the fire. Each profile was painstakingly researched and detailed to provide you with the information you need along the trail. So grab your copy today and get out in the great outdoors.

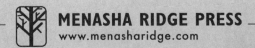

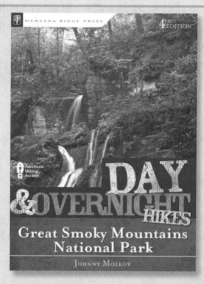
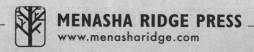

DEAR CUSTOMERS AND FRIENDS,

SUPPORTING YOUR INTEREST IN OUTDOOR ADVENTURE, travel, and an active lifestyle is central to our operations, from the authors we choose to the locations we detail to the way we design our books. Menasha Ridge Press was incorporated in 1982 by a group of veteran outdoorsmen and professional outfitters. For many years now, we've specialized in creating books that benefit the outdoors enthusiast.

Almost immediately, Menasha Ridge Press earned a reputation for revolutionizing outdoors- and travel-guidebook publishing. For such activities as canoeing, kayaking, hiking, backpacking, and mountain biking, we established new standards of quality that transformed the whole genre, resulting in outdoor-recreation guides of great sophistication and solid content. Menasha Ridge continues to be outdoor publishing's greatest innovator.

The folks at Menasha Ridge Press are as at home on a white-water river or mountain trail as they are editing a manuscript. The books we build for you are the best they can be, because we're responding to your needs. Plus, we use and depend on them ourselves.

We look forward to seeing you on the river or the trail. If you'd like to contact us directly, join in at www.trekalong.com or visit us at www.menasharidge.com. We thank you for your interest in our books and the natural world around us all.

SAFE TRAVELS,

Bob Sehlinger

BOB SEHLINGER
PUBLISHER